European School of Oncology

Monographs

Series Editor: U. Veronesi

A. B. Miller (Ed.)

Diet and the Aetiology of Cancer

Springer-Verlag Berlin Heidelberg New York
London Paris Tokyo

Professor Dr. ANTHONY B. MILLER
Department of Preventive Medicine and Biostatistics
University of Toronto
12 Queens Park Cres. West
4th Floor McMurrich Building
Toronto, Ontario M5S 1A8
Canada

The European School of Oncology gratefully acknowledges sponsorship for the Task Force on Diet and Cancer from Barilla S.p.A., Parma, Italy

ISBN 3-540-50681-0 Springer-Verlag Berlin Heidelberg New York
ISBN 0-387-50681-0 Springer-Verlag New York Berlin Heidelberg

Library of Congress Cataloging-in-Publication Data.
Diet and the aetiology of cancer. (Monographs / European School of Oncology) Bibliography: p. 1. Cancer–Nutritional aspects. 2. Cancer–Etiology. I. Miller, A. B. (Anthony B.) II. Series: Monographs (European School of Oncology)
RC268.45.D53 1989 616.99'4071 89-4060
ISBN 0-387-50681-0

Printing: Druckhaus Beltz, Hemsbach/Bergstr. Bookbinding: J. Schäffer GmbH & Co. KG, Grünstadt
2123/3145-543210

Foreword

The European School of Oncology came into existence to respond to a need for information, education and training in the field of the diagnosis and treatment of cancer. There are two main reasons why such an initiative was considered necessary. Firstly, the teaching of oncology requires a rigorously multidisciplinary approach which is difficult for the Universities to put into practice since their system is mainly disciplinary orientated. Secondly, the rate of technological development that impinges on the diagnosis and treatment of cancer has been so rapid that it is not an easy task for medical faculties to adapt their curricula flexibly.

With its residential courses for organ pathologies and the seminars on new techniques (laser, monoclonal antibodies, imaging techniques etc.) or on the principal therapeutic controversies (conservative or mutilating surgery, primary or adjuvant chemotherapy, radiotherapy alone or integrated), it is the ambition of the European School of Oncology to fill a cultural and scientific gap and, thereby, create a bridge between the University and Industry and between these two and daily medical practice.

One of the more recent initiatives of ESO has been the institution of permanent study groups, also called task forces, where a limited number of leading experts are invited to meet once a year with the aim of defining the state of the art and possibly reaching a consensus on future developments in specific fields of oncology.

The ESO Monograph series was designed with the specific purpose of disseminating the results of these study group meetings, and providing concise and updated reviews of the topic discussed.

It was decided to keep the layout relatively simple, in order to restrict the costs and make the monographs available in the shortest possible time, thus overcoming a common problem in medical literature: that of the material being outdated even before publication.

Umberto Veronesi
Chairman, Scientific Committee
European School of Oncology

Table of Contents

Introduction

A.B. Miller

Department of Preventive Medicine and Biostatistics, University of Toronto, Toronto, Ontario, M5S 1A8, Canada

The first meeting of the European School of Oncology Task Force on Diet, Nutrition and Cancer was held in March, 1988. In this monograph papers relating to the main presentations at the meeting are given, and at the end a summary of our main conclusions on the current scientific evidence on dietary factors in the aetiology of cancer.

Although several groups have issued dietary recommendations for the general population (sometimes described as "Interim Dietary Guidelines"), we did not feel that detailed consideration of possible recommendations was an appropriate task for our first meeting. We therefore concentrated on a review of the scientific evidence relating to the factors that seem largely to be associated with cancer risk, dietary fat (reviewed by Berrino, Hill and Wahrendorf) and fibre (reviewed by Jensen and Hill), but also considering other factors that can influence cancer risk (reviewed by Miller), of which one of the most important is alcohol consumption (reviewed by Jensen and Miller). In addition, an important paper by Riboli considers methodological issues in the investigation of diet and cancer in humans, issues that should be carefully considered by new investigators entering this field, but which can also be reviewed with profit by established investigators.

At the end of this first meeting, we commenced a detailed review of the ethical considerations that affect dietary recommendations; the quality of scientific evidence required in order to make recommendations for dietary change; the ways by which dietary change may be affected; the possibility that certain dietary changes might adversely affect the risk of some cancers and other diseases; the extent to which approaches to individuals at risk are feasible as distinct from mass population approaches; and the extent that cancer incidence could be reasonably expected to change following dietary recommendations, and the timing of such changes. We intend to continue our deliberations on these issues during our subsequent meetings, and include our conclusions in a second monograph on Diet, Nutrition and Cancer.

Dietary Fat, Nutritional Status and Endocrine-Associated Cancers

F. Berrino [1)], S. Panico [2)], P. Muti [1)]

1) Division of Epidemiology, Istituto Nazionale Tumori, Milano, Italy
2) Institute of Internal Medicine and Metabolic Diseases, Seconda Facoltà di Medicina, Università di Napoli, Italy

Introduction

The issue of dietary fats and hormone-dependent cancers of the reproductive organs seems far more complex today than a few years ago, when only a few analytical studies were available. Several studies that found an association are heavily flawed in the design and/or analysis, especially the earlier ones. Even well conducted studies, apparently, give contradictory results.

A number of theories are available which may explain the association between nutrition and hormonal status:

a) Nutrition affects steroid hormone metabolism through the enzymatic activity of adipose tissue: aromatase activity, which converts androgens into estrogens, mainly androstenedione to estrone [1]. Obese women, moreover, show a decreased production of 2-OH estrogen compounds, which could result in a relative hyperestrogenic state [2].

b) Fat in the diet affects enteric reabsorption of steroid hormones by influencing the intestinal flora [3].

c) Excess fat in the diet and obesity are associated with low levels of sex-hormone binding globulin and, therefore, with higher levels of free sex steroid hormones which would be available to target organs [4, 5].

d) Rich diet in young girls influences age at menarche, growth of hormone-dependent organs and, possibly, hormonal status in adulthood and age at menopause [6].

e) Excess fat in the diet and obesity increase the production of prolactin and other pituitary hormones [7].

A major problem in interpreting the role of diet in cancers of endocrine-dependent organs is that, with the exception of endometrial cancer, endocrine determinants are far from being clear. For breast cancer, for instance, a dozen hormonal hypotheses have been proposed [8, 9, 10], but a large number of hormonal studies have not solved the problem of which is the most plausible. Hormonal studies in prostatic and ovarian cancer have given conflicting results too. For endometrial cancer only, most of the empirical evidence points to a major aetiologic role of an estrogenic environment [11].

Most endocrine related cancers of the reproductive organs (we will consider breast, ovary, endometrium and prostate) are characterised by a higher incidence in wealthy occidental populations. Their incidence is heavily correlated, therefore, with indexes of food consumption such as per capita meat or fat [12]. Geographical studies, however, do not exclude the possibility that the high correlation may be attributable to the association of both fat in the diet and cancer incidence with other variables. We will focus here on the evidence derived from analytical studies carried out on individuals, e.g. cohort and case-control studies.

Breast Cancer

Mortality from breast cancer in different countries shows a strong correlation with the corresponding per capita consumption of fat [12, 13]. As the correlation coefficient is of the order of 0.9, theoretically fat could explain about 80% of the international variation in breast cancer mortality. The relationship, however, may be indirect, because countries with high fat consumption are distinctive in other respects as well, for example in gross national product [12].

The aetiological hypothesis linking dietary fat and breast cancer has been the object of many analytical observational studies which, inevitably, have not yielded identical results. A number of review articles are already available; however, they show a rather confusing pattern of inconsistent results. An overview of the issue in the light of Bradford-Hill's criteria for causal inference has recently been published [13]. Inconsistency seems to be the main obstacle to conclude a causal association between high dietary fat intake and breast cancer. A few studies have found a significant association with meat consumption [14-17], while others have not [18-21], or have shown only minor differences [22-24]. Most researchers who have looked at milk and/or dairy products have found at least some significant association [15-17,19,24,25], but one study did not find any [18]. A number of studies have shown an association with total fat consumption [24,26-29], at least a minor one [30,31], but others have not found any association [32,33] and a recent study [34] found a negative one.

Judgement on inconsistencies is not possible unless the validity of the studies is accurately evaluated. Although evaluation of published papers may be difficult if information on subjects, methods and material is poorly detailed, we have scrutinised each paper in order to judge whether the reported details of design and analysis offer sufficient evidence to exclude substantial information bias, selection bias, misclassification and confounding from uncontrolled variables. This procedure is bound to a certain amount of subjectivity, but we feel that it is possible to categorise papers according to different degrees of validity: those well designed and properly analyzed; those with one or more clearly identifiable major defects affecting their reliability; and those at an intermediate level.

Table 1. Analytical studies on diet and breast cancer

Year	1st Author	Design	No. of cases	Total or saturated fats	Meat	Milk & dairy	Vegetable fats	Fruit or vegetables
1987	Willett	P	601	na			na	
1988	Toniolo	N	250	+	sp	+	na	na
1978/85	Miller/Howe	N	400	+ *			- *	
1985	Hirohata	N,H	212	sp			sn	
1987	Hirohata	N,H	344	sp			na	
1986	Hislop	N	861		+ *	+ *		- *
1982	Kinlen	P	62		sp			
1988	Mills	P	186		na	na		
1986	Lubin F	N,H	818	+ *				sn *
1986/88	Katsouyanni	H	120		na	na		-
1982	Graham	H	2024	na				- *
1984	Talamini	H	368		na	+		
1986	Lé	H	1010			+		
1987	Jones	P	99	-			sn	
1978	Hirayama	P	139		+			
1978	Nomura	P	86		+	+		
1981	Lubin J	N	577		+	+		
1975	Philips	N,H	77		na	sp		
1985	Zemla	N	328		sp *			- *
1985	Sarin	H	68	+				

H = Hospital based case-control study
N = Case-control study with population or neighbouring controls
P = Cohort study
+ = Significant (p<0.05) positive association
sp = Suggestive of positive association
- = Significant (p<0.05) negative association
sn = Suggestive of negative association
na = No association
* = Association limited to subgroups

Table 1 summarises the results of 21 cohort or case-control studies relevant to the issue of dietary fat and breast cancer. They are ordered by the decreasing degree of reliability according to our judgement (and prejudice) on their design and analysis. The top third roughly corresponds to the studies we would rely upon without major uncertainties; the bottom third to those whose methodology section clearly reveals serious biases that prevent their use in a formal evaluation of the evidence; the middle third includes those papers on which one may raise some doubts but no formal fallacies could be identified. Our criteria to judge validity and to reject unreliable results are relatively simple and will be made clear by some examples.

Information bias should be considered in any case-control study that relies on interview data, but must be strongly suspected when cases and controls have been interviewed by different interviewers, or with different questionnaires, or in different seasons as in one Canadian study [16].

Information bias cannot be excluded even in prospective studies if information is collected when a sizeable fraction of the cases have already occurred. It is the case of a study in which the husband's diet was taken as a surrogate of the wife's exposure [15]. One may suspect such a bias also in the National Health and Nutrition Survey Follow-up Study (NHANES) [34], in which the prevalence of breast cancer at baseline was surprisingly low, about 1 per thousand, with respect to what one would expect [35].

Selection bias should always be suspected when hospital controls are used, especially if their disease may be related to dietary habits. This may be the case of orthopaedic [18-20] or gastrointestinal disorders [20,25,29] or of illnesses where probability of being treated in hospital is linked to social class (and social class is not controlled in the analysis) [20,25,33].

Insufficient data analysis points to a low degree of reliability, especially when substantial confounding can be hypothesized and is not adequately controlled: either because of absence of information, or because the categorization of potential confounders is vaguely described, or because they are clearly identifiable but not taken into account, as in the Japanese cohort study [14], in which the husband's occupation was strongly related both to breast cancer risk and to the frequency of meat consumption. Further examples are the NHANES [34], for which no control for race or cultural group is mentioned in the report, and a study on Hawaiian Japanese, in which education was a significant determinant of breast cancer risk not controlled in dietary analysis [15]. The commonly recognised constitutional and reproductive risk factors for breast cancer, on the contrary, do not seem to have any major confounding or modifying effect on the risks associated with dietary items.

Given the limited validity of dietary methods, some misclassification of fat consumption is unavoidable. This means that any risk difference is biased towards the null. On the other hand, whenever a strong association is found using methods which are grossly unreliable to categorise individuals, such as 24-hour recall [34], a major bias should be suspected. Other poor techniques include frequency interview questioning only a few food items [14,16,19,20,23]. Implausible observations such as very low caloric intake in the U.S. [34], or very high in India [28], also point to low validity of dietary assessment methods.

We have not included the study size in the criteria to define reliability. It clearly bears, however, in the weighing of evidence to reach valid inferences, not affected by the play of chance. In the table, therefore, we have indicated both the number of cases on which the analysis was based and the formal 5% significance when reached by the reported association.

The table shows that most results based on isolated questions on meat or milk products are heavily flawed, while those studies which tried to derive total fat intake from many sources are more reliable but still inconsistent. Those who show protection from fruits or vegetables belong to the intermediate reliability group.

Apparently the studies selected through our critical approach leave us with discrepancies as serious as those we had to face before. Now we have better reasons, however, to tentatively accept both negative and positive results as valid. The former allows us to reject the theory that any increase in fat consumption will increase breast cancer incidence. The latter requires admitting that there are instances in which an increase in fat consumption increases the risk. Along with these tentative acceptances comes the opportunity for formulating new theories and designing new studies susceptible of falsifying their predictions. Two theories have been proposed which might explain the inconsistencies on total fat consumption [36,37,38].

Firstly, different types of fats, namely fatty acid composition, may have different and even opposite effects. Secondly, an effect can be observed only within certain ranges of intake, or below a given level (e.g. up to about 50 g of total fat per day), so that in many Western populations no effect is detectable.

A recent reanalysis [27] of a Canadian study [26] suggests that saturated fatty acids increase the risk, while oleic acid, the intake of which, however, is heavily correlated with the former, is protective.

A recent case-control study carried out in Northern Italy, based on dietary history and characterised by a high compliance of both incident cases and population controls, shows a significant increase of risk with increasing total and saturated fat consumption up to a level roughly corresponding to the median intake and no To challenge these theories further studies should be carried out in populations with a wide variety of fat intake and focus on fatty acid composition of diet and/or some biological indicator of the same (e.g. red blood cell membrane or adipose tissue composition).

The judgement procedure we have adopted, which has resulted in a review on dietary fat and breast cancer [39], is certainly affected by our prejudices and methodological beliefs. Also the interpretation of a study result, whether positive or negative, in absence of statistical significance, is highly subjective. Even if shaped on some prejudices and beliefs, however, thorough criticism helps in concentrating on the most reliable results, instead of just listing inconsistencies, for stimulating alternative hypotheses and devising crucial observations.

Table 2 summarises the results of 21 studies [14,19,40-58] reporting on the association between some anthropometric measurements and risk of breast cancer. Overweight has been rather consistently found associated with breast cancer in postmenopausal but not in premenopausal women. The usual interpretation of this finding refers to the endocrine activity of adipose tissue [1]. Height has been frequently found positively associated with breast cancer in postmenopausal women. This might be explained by nutritional patterns influencing growth in childhood and adolescence.

Cancer of the Endometrium

Endometrial cancer is positively correlated in ecological studies [12,59] with per capita fat consumption, with coefficients of the same order of magnitude as for breast cancer.

Any condition that raises the levels of endogenous or exogenous estrogens (in absence of contemporaneous rise of progestogens) apparently enhances endometrial cancer risk [11]. Obesity is one such condition. Heavy body weight or various body mass indexes have been consistently identified in many studies as strong risk factors [54, 60-67]. The large American Cancer Society prospective study on 419,060 women followed up from 1959 to 1972 [54] shows a significant increase of endometrial cancer mortality with increase in body weight (from unity among women weighing below the height specific average to RR = 1.36 for those weighing 10-19% more, RR = 1.85 for 20-29%, RR = 2.30 for 30-39%, to RR = 5.42 for women weighing 40% or more above the average). Higher RRs have been found for premenopausal women [66,67].

Obesity is obviously linked to diet but the role of diet independent of its effect on nutritional status has not yet been thoroughly studied. Death rates for endometrial cancer are lower than expected among Californian Seventh-day Adventists [20] who tend to be lacto-ovo-vegetarians. Since their overall level of fat intake is not appreciably different from non-vegetarians, meat-derived fats seem more likely to be of aetiologic importance. Body weight, though, was not considered in this study.

Table 2. Studies on nutritional status and breast cancer

						Premenopausal				Postmenopausal				All			
Ref.	Author	Country	Year	(a) Design	(b) Method	Weight	Height	(c) BMI	Others	Weight	Height	BMI	Others	Weight	Height	BMI	Others
40	Valaoras	G	1969	H	n.i. (d)									+	+	+	
41	Lin	RC	1971	H	n.i.	sp				+				+	na		
42	Mirra	BR	1971	H	n.i. (d)	na	na	na		+	sp	+					
43	Stazewsky	PL	1978	H	n.i.									+			
44	Ravhinar	YU	1972	H	n.i.									na	sp		
45	Stavraky	CN	1974	H	n.i.			sn				na					
46	de Waard	NL	1974	P	M					+	+	na	+ (e)				
47	Herity	IRL	1975	H	M										na		
48/49	de Waard	NL	75/77	P	M	sn	sp	sn	sn (e)	+	+	na	+ (e)				
49	de Waard	J	1977	H	n.i.	+	+			+	+						
50	Adami	S	1977	P	M	na	na	na	na (f)	na	na	na	na (f)				
51	Soini	SF	1977	H	n.i.									na	na	na	na (g)
52	Wynder	US	1978	H	M (h)	na	na	na		na	na	na					
53	Choi	CN	1978	P	n.i.	- (i)	na			+ (k)	sp						
14	Hirayama	J	1978	H	n.i.	sp				+	sp			+	sp		
14	id.	id.	id.	P	n.i.									+	sp		
54	Lew	US	1979	P	R												+ (l)
55	Helmrich	US	1983	H	n.i.			-				+					
19	Talamini	I	1984	H	n.i. (d)			sp				+				+	
56	Lubin	IL	1985	H	R (d)			sn				+ (k)		na	na		sp (e)
57	Willet	US	1985	P	R (d)	-	na	-									
58	La Vecchia	I	1987	H	n.i. (d)			+				sp					

+ = Significantly positive ($p<0.05$) association
- = Significantly negative ($p<0.05$) association
sp = Suggestive of positive association
sn = Suggestive of negative association
na = No association

(a) : P = Population based; H = Hospital based study
(b) : M = Direct measure R = Reported measure n.i. = Not indicated
(c) : Body Mass Index (Quetelet index) = Weight/Height squared
(d) : Adjusted for education and reproductive factors
(e) : Body surface
(f) : Broca's index = 100 Weight/0.9 (Height-100)
(g) : Weight x Height and breast size
(h) : Only height was measured
(i) : Both for present and past weight
(k) : Particularly in older women
(l) : % of height specific average weight

In a hospital-based study carried out in Italy, cases and controls were asked to judge if their consumption of butter, margarine and oil was low, intermediate, or high [68]. No clear trend was evident for any single item, but a significantly positive trend became evident when an overall index of intake was derived summing up the three scores.

Cancer of the Prostate

International comparisons revealed a striking difference between diet in high and low-risk areas for prostate cancer [69]. Fat intake accounted for up to 40% of daily calories in the high-risk areas and 20% of calories in low-risk ones.
Heavy body weight has also been found to be associated with prostatic cancer [54,70], but not consistently [69,72,77[(Table 3). The positive studies include two prospective studies [54,70]. The American Cancer Society study [54] shows RRs of 1.4 and 1.3, respectively, for men weighing 20-29% and 30% more than the desirable weight. With one exception, a Japanese cohort study [71], all the analytical studies of diet and prostatic cancer (one cohort [70] and six case-control studies [72-76]) find at least some association with total fat indices and/or with consumption of one or more food items of animal origin and rich in fat (meat, eggs, milk or dairy products). The observed RRs are in the range of 1.5 to 3.0. One must consider that all these studies were based on rather rough dietary indicators (few questions on daily or weekly frequency of a few food items). In these conditions random misclassification is likely to occur. The magnitude of the association, therefore, may be larger than the one observed.
The inconsistency of the Japanese results, which do not show any association with meat intake, are not easy to explain; perhaps an association can be observed only for high levels of meat intake, which in Japan is relatively infrequent.
A few of these studies were analysed in rather a crude way. Others duly took account of both age and socio-economic indicators in the analysis [70,72,73]. The prospective study on Adventists [70] also adjusts for weight and for the other food items. None take into account other suspected risk factors for prostatic cancer, such as sexual behaviour.

Table 3. Diet, body weight and prostatic cancer

1st Author	Year	Design	Fat Indices	Meat	Eggs	Milk & Dairy	Overweight
Snowdon	1984	P		sp	sp	sp	+
Hirayama	1979	P		na		na	
Graham	1983	H	+	+			na
Kolonel	1983	N	+ (1)				
Hesmat	1985	H	sp (2)				
Meikel (3)	1982	H			+	+	+
Shuman	1982	HN		na (4)	sp	+	
Rotkin	1977	H		sp	+	+	
Lew	1979	P					+
Wynder	1971	H					na
Greenwald	1974	P					na

(1) : Positive trend over 70 years only (significance of trend not stated)
(2) : For consumption under 50 years only
(3) : Cited by Snowdon [70]
(4) : Chicken and fish protective
\+ = Significant ($p<0.05$) association
na = No association
sp = Suggestive of positive association
H = Hospital based case-control study
N = Case-control study with population or neighbouring controls
P = Cohort study

The hormonal mechanism by which excess fat in the diet and obesity influences prostatic cancer is not known, but there are indications that diet may alter the hormonal metabolism in men [74]. When South African black males were fed a Western diet, isocaloric with the African diet but supplying 40% of calories from fat and 70% of protein from animal sources, the urinary estrogens and androgens were significantly increased. American black and white males, when fed a vegetarian diet, showed a decrease in urinary estrogens and androgens [78].

Cancer of the Ovary

Ovarian cancer shows a similar geographical correlation to that for endometrial and breast cancer [12,59] but the empirical evidence available on diet and ovarian cancer, unfortunately, is rather confusing. There are no large prospective studies. Californian Adventists [79] have a lower incidence than non-Adventists, but factors other than diet, e.g. reproductive life and weight, might account for the difference. Vegetarian nuns in the U.K. [22] have the same risk as single women, but the study is small and the nuns may have other reasons for being at risk. Two case-control studies gave opposite results on both fat in the diet and body weight [80,81]. Both adjust for the major determinants of ovarian cancer, i.e., age and parity. The American Cancer Society prospective study on body weight [54] showed a significant excess of ovarian cancer death (RR = 1.63) only for women weighing 40% more for the height specific average.

Table 4. Fat diet, body weight and ovarian cancer

1st Author	Year	Design	Fat rich Diet	Over-weight
Byers	1983	H	na	- (1)
Cramer	1984	H	+	sp
Kinlen	1982	P	na	
Snowdon	1983 (2)	P	+	
Lew	1979	P		+

P = Prospective study
H = Hospital based case-control study
1 = Over 50 yrs only
2 = Cited in Thomas and Chu [59]
\+ = Significantly positive ($p<0.05$) association
\- = Significantly negative ($p<0.05$) association
na = No association
sp = Suggestive of positive association

Conclusions

Epidemiological studies have provided some evidence that dietary fats are a determinant of breast cancer. The association is not a simple linear one. There may be no exposure-effect relationship at high levels of intake and a number of observations suggest that fatty acid composition is important. Experimental data in rodents are consistent with the positive epidemiological observations. Obesity is associated with increased risk of breast cancer in postmenopausal but not premenopausal women. One must consider, however, that the causes of breast cancer are mostly unknown and that some unidentified confounder might partially explain these associations.

There is some evidence that prostatic cancer is associated with high intake of foods rich in animal fat. The issue should be addressed with larger studies and more reliable dietary assessment methods.

Obesity is a determinant of endometrial cancer, most probably a causal one, but there is no information to discriminate between the role of dietary fats and other calorie-providing nutrients.

There is insufficient information to make any inference on diet, obesity and ovarian cancer.

REFERENCES

1 Edman CD, MacDonald PC: Effect of obesity on conversion of plasma androstenedione to estrone in ovulatory and anovulatory young women. Am J Obstet Gynecol 1978 (130):456-460
2 Schneider S, Fishmann J: Effects of obesity on estradiol metabolism: decreased formation of nonuterotropic metabolites. J Clin Endocrinol Metab 1983 (56):973-978
3 Gorbach SL: Estrogens, breast cancer and intestinal flora. Rev Infect Dis 1984 (6, suppl 1):85-90
4 Armstrong BK, Brown JB, Clarke HT et al: Diet and reproductive hormones: a study of vegetarian and non-vegetarian postmenopausal women. JNCI 1981 (67):761-767
5 Ingram DM, Bennett FC, Willcox D, de Klerk N: Effect of low-fat diet on female sex hormone levels. JNCI 1987 (79):1225-1229
6 Hill P, Wynder EL, Garbaczewski L, Helman P, Hill M, Sporangisa J, Huskisson J: Diet and menarche in different ethnic groups. Eur J Cancer 1980 (16):519-525
7 Hill P, Wynder EL: Diet and prolactin release. Lancet 1976 (2):800-807
8 Zumoff B: Hormone profiles and the epidemiology of breast cancer. In: Stoll BA (ed) Endocrine Relationships in Breast Cancer. William Heinemann Med Books, London 1982 pp 3-47
9 Moore JW, Thomas BS, Wang DY: Endocrine status of breast cancer. Cancer Surv 1986 (5):536-559
10 Berrino F, Muti P, Pisani P: Overview of the etiological hypotheses linking endogenous steroid hormones and breast cancer. Meeting on Prospective Studies on Diet and Cancer. IARC, Lyon 1987 (in press)
11 Henderson BE, Ross R, Bernstein L: Estrogens as a cause of human cancer: The Richard and Hinda Rosenthal Foundation Award Lecture. Cancer Res 1988 (48):246-253
12 Armstrong B, Doll R: Environmental factors and cancer incidence and mortality in different countries with special reference to dietary practices. Int J Cancer 1975 (15):617-631
13 Goodwin PJ, Boyd NF: Critical appraisal of the evidence that dietary fat intake is related to breast cancer risk in humans. JNCI 1987 (79):473-485
14 Hirayama T: Epidemiology of breast cancer with special reference to the role of diet. Prev Med 1978 (7):173-195
15 Nomura A, Henderson BE, Lee J: Breast cancer and diet among the Japanese in Hawaii. Am J Clin Nutr 1978 (31):2020-2025
16 Lubin JH, Burns PE, Blot WJ, Ziegler RG, Lees AW, Fraumeni JF Jr: Dietary factors and breast cancer risk. Int J Cancer 1981 (28):685-689
17 Hislop TG, Coldman AJ, Elwood JM, Braner G, Kan L: Childhood and recent eating patterns and risk of breast Cancer. Cancer Detect Prev 1986 (9):47-58
18 Katsouyanni K, Trichopoulos D, Boyle P, Xirouchaki E, Trichopoulos A, Lisseos B, Vasilaros S, MacMahon B: Diet and breast cancer: A case-control study in Greece. Int J Cancer 1986 (38):815-820
19 Talamini R, La Vecchia C, De Carli A, Franceschi S, Grattoni E, Grigoletto E, Liberati A, Tognoni G: Social factors, diet and breast cancer in a Northern Italian population. Br J Cancer 1984 (49):723-729
20 Phillips R L: role of lifestyle and dietary habits in risk of cancer among Seventh-day Adventist. Cancer Res 1975 (35):3513-3522
21 Mills PK, Annegers JF, Phillips RL: Animal product consumption and subsequent fatal breast cancer risk among Seventh-day Adventists. Am J Epidemiol 1988 (127):440-453
22 Kinlen LJ: Meat and fat consumption and cancer mortality: A study of strict religious order in Britain. Lancet 1982 (1):946-949
23 Zemla B: The role of selected dietary elements in breast cancer risk among native and migrant populations in Poland. Nutr Cancer 1985 (6):187-190
24 Toniolo PG, Riboli E, Protta F, Charrel M, Cappa APM: Calorie-providing nutrients and risk of breast cancer. To be published
25 Lé MG, Moulton LH, Hill C, Kramar A: Consumption of dairy produce and alcohol in a case-control study of breast cancer. JNCI 1986 (77):633-636
26 Miller AB, Kelly A, Choi NW, Matthews V, Morgan RW, Munan L, Burch JD, Feather J, Howe GR, Jain M: A study of diet and breast cancer. Am J Epidemiol 1978 (107):499-509
27 Howe GR: The use of polytomous dual response data to increase power in case-control studies: an application to the association between dietary fat and breast cancer. J Chron Dis 1985 (38):663-670
28 Sarin R, Tandon RK, Paul S, Kapur GBML, Kapur K: Diet, body fat and plasma lipids in breast cancer. Indian J Med Res 1985 (81):493-498
29 Lubin F, Wax Y, Modan B: Role of fat, animal protein and dietary fiber in breast cancer etiology: a case-control study. JNCI 1986 (77):605-612
30 Hirohata T, Shigematsu T, Nomura A, Nomura MY, Horie A, Hirohata I: Occurrence of breast cancer in relation to diet and reproductive history: a case-control study in Fukuoka, Japan. Natl Cancer Inst Monogr. 1985 (69):187-190
31 Hirohata T, Nomura AMY, Hankin JH, Kolonel LN, Lee J: An epidemiologic study on the association between diet and breast cancer. JNCI 1987 (78):595-600
32 Willett W C, Stampfer M J, Colditz G A, Rosner B A, Hennekens CH, Speizer FE: Dietary fat and the risk of breast cancer. N Engl J Med 1987 (316):22-28
33 Graham S, Marshall J, Mettlin C, Rzepka T, Nemoto T, Byers T: Diet in the epidemiology of breast cancer. Am J Epidemiol 1982 (116):68-75
34 Jones YD, Schatakin A, Green SB, Block G, Brinton L, Ziegler RG, Hoover R, Taylor DR: Dietary fat and breast cancer in the national health and nutrition examination survey.I Epidemiologic follow-up study. JNCI 1987 (79):465-471
35 Feldman AR, Kessler L, Myers MH, Naughton MD: The prevalence of cancer-estimates based on the Connecticut tumor registry. N Engl J Med 1986 (315):1394-1397
36 Carroll KK, Braden LM, Bell JR, Kalamegham R: Fat and cancer. Cancer 1986 (58):1818-1825

37 Wynder EL, Rose DP, Cohen LA: Diet and breast cancer in causation and therapy. Cancer 1986 (58):1804-1813
38 Potter JD: letter, N Engl J Med 1987 (317) p 166
39 Panico S, Muti P, Berrino F: Grassi alimentari e cancro della mammella: le ipotesi, i meccanismi e l'evidenza epidemiologica. Argomenti di Oncologia 1988 (9):65-79
40 Valaoras VG, MacMahon B, Trichopoulos D, Polychronopoulou A: Lactation and reproductive histories of breast cancer patients in greater Athens 1965-1967. Int J Cancer 1969 (4):350-363
41 Lin T M, Chen KP, MacMahon B: Epidemiologic characteristics of cancer of the breast in Taiwan. Cancer 1971 (27):1497-1504
42 Mirra AP, Cole P, MacMahon B: Breast cancer in an area of high parity: Sao Paolo, Brazil. Cancer Res 1971 (31):77-83
43 Stazewsky J: Unpublished data cited by Wynder [52]
44 Ravnihar B, MacMahon B, Lindtner J: Epidemiologic features of breast cancer in Slovenia, 1965 -1967. Europ J Cancer 1971 (7):295-306
45 Stavraky K, Emmons S: Breast cancer in premenopausal and postmenopausal women. JNCI 1974 (53):647-654
46 de Waard F, Baanders-van Halewijn EA: A prospective study in general practice on breast cancer risk in postmenopausal women. Int J Cancer 1974 (14):153-160
47 Herity BA, O'Halloran MJ, Bourke GJ, Wilson-Davis K: A study of breast cancer in Irish women. Brit J Prev Soc Med 1975 (29):178-181
48 de Waard F: Breast cancer incidence and nutritional status with particular reference to body weight and height. Cancer Res 1975 (35):3351-3356
49 de Waard F, Cornelis JP, Aoki K, Yoshida M: Breast cancer incidence according to weight and height in two cities of the Netherlands and in Aichi prefecture, Japan. Cancer 1977 (40):1269-1275
50 Adami HO, Rimsten A, Stenkvist B, Vegelius J: Influence of height, weight and obesity on risk of breast cancer in an unselected Swedish population. Br J Cancer 1977 (36):787-792
51 Soini I: Risk factors of breast cancer in Finland. Int J Epidemiol 1977 (6):365-373
52 Wynder EL, MacCornack FA, Stellman SD: The epidemiology of breast cancer in 785 United States Caucasian women. Cancer 1978 (41):2341-2354
53 Choi NW, Howe GR, Miller AB, Matthews V, Morgan RW, Munan L, Burch JD, Feather J, Jain M, Kelly A: An epidemiologic study of breast cancer. Am J Epidemiol 1978 (107):510-521
54 Lew EA, Garfinkel L: Variations in mortality by weight among 750,000 men and women. J Chron Dis 1979 (32):563-576
55 Helmrich SP, Shapiro S, Rosenberg L, Kaufman DW, Slone D, Bain C, Miettinen OS, Stolley PD, Rosenshein NB, Knapp RC, Leavitt T Jr, Schottenfeld D, Engle RL, Levy M: Risk factors for breast cancer. Am J Epidemiol 1983 (117):35-45
56 Lubin F, Ruder AM, Wax Y, Modan B: Overweight and changes in weight throughout adult life in breast cancer etiology. Am J Epidemiol 1985 (122):579-588
57 Willett WC, Browne ML, Bain C, Lipnick RJ, Stampfer MJ, Rosner B, Colditz GA, Hennekens CH, Speizer FE: Relative weight and risk of breast cancer among premenopausal women. Am J Epidemiol 1985 (122):731-740
58 La Vecchia C, Decarli A, Parazzini F, Gentile A, Negri E, Cecchetti G, Franceschi S: General Epidemiology of breast cancer in Northern Italy. Int J Epidemiol 1987 (16):347-355
59 Thomas DB, Chu J: Nutritional and endocrine factors in reproductive organ cancers: Opportunities for primary prevention. J Chron Dis 1986 (12):1031-1050
60 Hertig AT, Sommers SC: Genesis of endometrial carcinoma 1. Study of prior biopsies. Cancer 1949 (2):946-956
61 Stewart HL, Dunham LJ, Casper I, Dorn HF, Thomas LB, Edgomb JH, Symeonidis A: Epidemiology of cancers of the uterine cervix and corpus, breast and ovary in Israel and New York City. JNCI 1966 (37):1-95
62 Wynder EL, Escher GC, Mantel N: An epidemiological investigation of cancer of the endometrium. Cancer 1966 (19):489-520
63 Elwood JM, Cole P, Rothman KJ, Kaplan SD: Epidemiology of endometrial cancer. JNCI 1977 (59):1055-1060
64 Schenker JG, Tal J: Adenocarcinoma of the endometrium in Israel, 1960-1968. Cancer 1980 (46):2752-2758
65 Kelsey JL, LiVolsi VA, Holford TR, Fischer DB, Mostow ED, Schwartz PE, O'Connor T, White C: A case-control study of endometrial cancer. Am J Epidemiol 1982 (116):333-342
66 Henderson BE, Casagrande JT, Pike MC, Mack T, Rosario I, Duke A: The epidemiology of endometrial cancer in young women. Brit J Cancer 1983 (47):749-756
67 La Vecchia C, Franceschi S, Decarli A, Gallus G, Tognoni G: Risk factors for endometrial cancer at different ages. JNCI 1984 (73):667-671
68 La Vecchia C, Decarli A, Fasoli M, Gentile A: Nutrition and diet in the etiology of endometrial cancer. Cancer 1986 (57):1248-1253
69 Wynder EL, Mabuchi K, Whitmore WF: Epidemiology of cancer of the prostate. Cancer 1971 (28):344-360
70 Snowdon DA, Phillips RL, Choi W: Diet, obesity, and risk of fatal prostate cancer. Am J Epidemiol 1984 (120):244-250
71 Hirayama T: Epidemiology of prostate cancer with special reference to the role of diet. Natl Cancer Inst Monogr 1979 (53):149-155
72 Graham S, Haughey B, Marshall J, Priore R, Byers T, Rzepka T, Mettlin C, Pontes J E: Diet in the epidemiology of carcinoma of the prostate gland. JNCI 1983 (70):687-692
73 Kolonel LN, Nomura AMY, Ward Hinds M, Hirohata T, Hankin J H, Lee J: Role of diet in cancer incidence in Hawaii. Cancer Res 1983 (Supp.43):2397-2402
74 Heshmat MY, Kaul L, Kovi J, Jackson MA, Jackson AG, Jones GW, Edson M, Enterline JP, Worrell RG, Perry SL: Nutrition and prostate cancer: A case-control study. The Prostate 1985 (6):7-17
75 Schuman LM, Mandel JS, Radke A, Seal U, Halberg F: Some selected features of the epidemiology of

prostatic cancer: Minneapolis-St. Paul, Minnesota case-control study, 1976-1979. In: Magnus K (ed) Trends in Cancer Incidence: Causes and Practical Implications. Washington DC: Hemisphere Press 1982 pp 345-354
76 Rotkin ID: Studies in the epidemiology of prostatic cancer: Expanded sampling. Cancer Treat Rep 1977 (61):173-180
77 Greenwald P, Damon A, Kirmss V, Polan AK: Physical and demographic features of men before developing cancer of the prostate. JNCI 1974 (53):341-346
78 Hill P, Wynder EL, Garbaczewski L, Garnes H, Walker ARP: Diet and urinary steroids in black and white North American men and black South African men. Cancer Res 1979 (39):5101-5105
79 Snowdon DA, Phillips RL: Diet and reproductive factors and fatal ovarian cancer. Abstract presented at the 16th Annual Meeting of the Society for Epidemiologic Research, 15-17 June 1983, Winnipeg, Canada
80 Byers T, Marshall J, Graham S, Mettlin C, Swanson M: A case-control study of dietary and nondietary factors in ovarian cancer. JNCI 1983 (71):681-686
81 Cramer DW, Welch WR, Hutchison G B, Willett W, Scully RE: Dietary animal fat in relation to ovarian cancer risk. Obstet Gynecol 1984 (63):833-838

Dietary Fat, Dietary Cholesterol and Obesity as Risk Factors for Colorectal Cancer, Kidney Cancer and Other Tumours

J. Wahrendorf

Institute of Epidemiology and Biometry, German Cancer Research Center, 6900 Heidelberg, Federal Republic of Germany

Introduction

While a role of nutrition in human carcinogenesis is generally accepted, the identification of specific dietary components responsible for it, the quantitative nature of their involvement, and the detailed mechanism behind it is not yet identified or remains an area of debate. Dietary fat is probably one of the most intensively discussed and investigated components in this framework and it may be that the role of dietary fat in the aetiology of coronary heart diseases has contributed to this orientation of research efforts.

The epidemiological and medical literature, both on an international level and in some national, non-English language journals or monographs, is full of review articles or chapters on diet and cancer and related issues. One gets the impression that there are more review articles than original papers or studies. This predominance of review articles explains the high expectations of the scientific and non-scientific community in this question as well as the great problems in accumulating new compelling evidence through recognizable studies. The various review articles at hand [1-11], and only few are cited here for reasons of space, are markedly similar and the authors' interpretations may deviate only in small nuances.

Evidence for the role of dietary fat in human carcinogenesis can come from various sources. Experimental studies investigate putative risk factors in specially established experimental systems (chemical-induced organ-specific models for carcinogenesis in rodents) and provide interesting clues about possible mechanisms. However, firm evidence about cancer risk for humans associated with dietary habits can only come from epidemiological observations. Different types of observational studies contribute in this respect.

Although descriptive epidemiological studies and correlation studies are usually considered not to supply much evidence on the causality of a risk factor for the occurrence of cancer, the situation is particularly interesting in the case of dietary fat and colon cancer. There are many such studies which demonstrate a correlation between per capita intake of dietary fat and colon cancer incidence or colon cancer mortality in different countries. While some studies find a clear-cut correlation between per capita intake of dietary fat and colon cancer incidence and mortality in different countries [12-15], other studies conducted on a national level or within a smaller number of countries and including secular trends report no clear evidence for such a correlation between dietary fat consumption and colon cancer risk [16-18]. Comparison of colon cancer risk in different ethnic groups or groups of dietary-related religious practices also shows no clear picture concerning a possible role of dietary fat in the aetiology of colorectal cancer [19-21].

There remain essential problems in the interpretation of correlation studies between countries in relation to per capita intake statistics and cancer incidence or mortality statistics. Most important of all, the essential question, i.e., do those who eat fat get cancer or not, remains unanswered with such approaches. The large variation of per capita intake of dietary fat between countries encountered in such correlation studies does not materialize in within-country correlation studies and neither in within-country cohort or case-control studies. The greater homogeneity of dietary habits within one country makes it difficult to detect specific foods or nutrients explaining a gradient in cancer incidence or mortality.

Other dietary components such as meat or protein are often associated with high fat consumption and show in the above-mentioned correlation studies strong positive associations when compared between countries, but similarly conflicting evidence when analysed within countries with respect to their correlation with colorectal cancer incidence and mortality.

In one study [22] the mortality of colon cancer was correlated simultaneously to per capita intake of dietary fat, dietary cholesterol and fibre. The exposure information related to time periods about 10 years before that of mortality statistics. Partial correlations were most pronounced for dietary cholesterol when controlling for dietary fat and fibre but not vice versa.

Metabolic studies investigating dietary and faecal characteristics of random samples from populations with different risks of colorectal cancer have been conducted, mainly comparing Japanese, North American and Scandinavian populations [23-25]. Although measurements of some metabolic parameters such as faecal bile acid concentrations, which may relate to dietary fat intake (and fibre intake) were in parallel to gradients of risk in colorectal cancer, these studies did not show any consistent differences concerning dietary fat intake itself.

Case-control Studies on Colorectal Cancer and Dietary Fat and/or Dietary Cholesterol

In a large case-control study in two Canadian cities, 348 cases of cancer of the colon and 194 cases of cancer of the rectum were individually matched by age, sex and neighbourhood of residence, to 554 population controls, and frequency matched to 535 hospital controls who had undergone abdominal operations. Detailed dietary history interviews were conducted for all study participants and analysed in relation to specific nutrients, food items and food groups [26,27]. Consumption of saturated fat was found to be associated with an increased risk of colorectal cancer. The relative risk gradients along tertiles of the distributions of saturated fat consumption in males and females span ranges from unity to about 2.0. There were nutrients highly correlated with saturated fat (calories, total protein, total fat, oleic acid and cholesterol) which showed also significant risk gradients. Food items correlated to saturated fat intake showed a reduced ability to describe the relative risk gradient. The authors concluded that the evidence is most suggestive for saturated fat intake being the important risk factor.

Other case-control studies [28-34] investigated the consumption of high-fat foods as a risk factor for colorectal cancer. Some studies reported an increased risk associated with intake of these foods, although these associations did not always reach statistical significance. Other studies were negative in this respect [31,32]. In other studies [33,34], particular food items such as meat consumption showed an association with colorectal cancer risk.

In a large case-control study on colorectal cancer in Australia with more than 700 cases and a similar number of controls [35], an increased relative risk of 1.4 for dietary fat intake was reported. This estimate refers to different categories of increased fat intake in males and in females and was significant after adjustment for meat and vegetable intake.

In a case-control study from southern France [36], cases reported a lower consumption of oil than controls, but no effect was found for a specific effect of dietary fat intake on colorectal cancer risk.

A population-based investigation in Adelaide (Australia) [37], by studying 419 cases of colorectal cancer and 732 controls, found an increased risk with increased energy intake or protein consumption, while the risk associated with dietary fat intake was not consistently elevated.

In the analysis of a case-control study from Utah [38], the close association of dietary fat with total energy intake led to the finding that the colorectal cancer risk was most clearly

associated with total energy intake; when controlled for this, the effect of dietary fat - though elevated - appeared to be not significant.
No effect of dietary fat nor total energy or protein was found in a case-control study in Belgium [39]. A small study in one clinic in the Federal Republic of Germany showed a non-significantly higher intake of dietary fat in cases [40].
The results of all these case-control studies are summarized in Table 1.
Many of the above-mentioned studies have also investigated other components of diet, in particular dietary fibre. Depending on the method of analysis, some of these studies reported that high consumption of dietary fat associated with low consumption of dietary fibre is associated with colon cancer risk [29], or found such indications for related food groups [33].

Studies on Adenomatous Polyps

In a few case-control studies [41-42], cases of adenomatous polyps were considered. While one study [41] showed a higher consumption of fat among male cases compared to healthy controls, no effect of dietary fat intake was seen in the second study [42].

Cohort Studies in Relation to Dietary Fat and Dietary Cholesterol

Cohort studies reported in the recent past and initiated some 10 or 20 years ago are faced with the problem of the methodology of dietary assessment applied initially. When compared with recently developed standards [43,44], these methodologies make the results sometimes difficult to interprete.
In one cohort study an inverse relationship of saturated fat intake to colon cancer risk was reported [45], while in another study, also conducted among Japanese population groups [46], a protective effect of meat consumption against colorectal cancer mortality was reported. Another study [47] did not find any association between dietary fat intake or related nutrients and colon cancer risk. In a study conducted on Seventh-Day Adventists [48], some food items (consumption of eggs or coffee) as well as obesity turned out to be significantly related to colon cancer mortality. However, no clear indication of an effect of dietary fat intake can be derived from these findings.
In an ongoing cohort study with 90,000 American nurses the risk of colorectal cancer was found to be elevated with increasing dietary fat intake, particularly saturated and monounsaturated fat but not polyunsaturated fat [49].
In a very large cohort study of the American Cancer Society conducted among 750,000 men and women, an excess mortality of colorectal cancer was found among males who were 40% or more overweight [50].

Kidney cancer

Correlations between per capita fat intake and renal cancer mortality [51], together with the frequent observation from case-control studies that obesity is associated with an increased risk of renal cancer incidence or mortality, lead to the hypothesis that dietary fat and cholesterol intake may be associated with the occurrence of this cancer. All studies which particularly investigated the role of obesity [52-55], found a clear-cut effect, frequently in both sexes, for this risk factor. Table 2 summarizes the elevated relative risk estimates between the extreme categories of the body mass index scale. It should be noted that in some studies [55] the intermediate categories were not associated with an increased risk.
When analysing for dietary components the intake of dietary protein or related foods has been found to be positively associated with the risk of renal cell cancer [56,57]. These findings, though not particularly pointing to a specific role of dietary fat and/or cholesterol, neverthelesss are consistent with the hypothesis that a high intake of fat or cholesterol in conjunction with their metabolic interaction with smoking and hormones can play a role in human renal cell carcinogenesis.

Table 1. Summary of findings in relation to dietary fat intake from case-control studies on colorectal cancer

Study area and period	Reference	Number of cases and controls a)	Source of controls b)	Dietary method c)	Summary of results
Canada 1976-1978	[26,27]	542; 1077 C:348; R:194	H, N	DH	increased risk with increasing consumption of total fat or saturated fat
Japan	[28]	157; 307 C:69; R:88	H	Q	no association with dietary fat intake
USA 1959-1964	[32]	791; 409 C:468; R:323	H	Q	no association with dietary fat intake
USA 1973-1976	[29]	99; 280	H	F	non-sigificant increase in comsumption of high-fat foods in cases
USA 1970-1977	[30]	86; 176 C:58; R:28	H	F	increased risk with high consumption of meat and dairy products
Israel 1967-1969	[31]	295; 510 C:198; R:77	H, N	F	no association with dietary fat intake
Hawaii (Japanese) 1966-1970	[34]	179; 307	H	F	no association with dietary fat intake, but with meat intake
Greece 1979-1980	[33]	100; 100	H	F	association with meat intake
Australia 1980 - d)	[35]	715; 727 C:392; R:323	C	DH	increased risk for dietary fat intake
Australia 1979-1980	[37]	419; 732 C:220; R:323	C	QF	increased risk with energy intake and protein, no consistent effect for dietary fat
France 1979-1984	[36]	399; 399 C:196; R:153 e)	H	DH	no association with dietary fat intake
USA 1976-1978	[38]	246; 484 C: 246	C	DH	increased risk with increasing total energy consumption, no independent effect of dietary fat
Belgium 1978-1983	[39]	818; 2851 C:453; R:365	C	DH	no association with dietary fat intake
Fed.Rep Germany 1976-1977	[40]	49; 60 C:49	H	P	insignificantly increased intake of dietary fat in cases

a) C: colon; R: rectum

b) H: hospital controls; N: neighbourhood controls; C: community or population controls

c) DH: diet history; Q: questionnaire not specified; F: food frequency questionnaire; QF: quantitative food frequency questionnaire; P: dietary protocol (6 days)

d) ascertainment period of controls not specified

e) 36 cancers of rectosigmoid junction, 5 multiple and 9 unspecified localisations.

Table 2. Relative risk estimates for increased kidney cancer risk between extreme body mass index (BMI) categories

Reference	Number of BMI categories	Relative risk for highest compared to lowest category Males	Females
[52]	2	2.8	2.1
[53]	3	2.7	2.4
[54]	4	1.3	2.3
[55]	5	2.5	2.6

Other cancers

Besides colorectal cancer, kidney cancer and endocrine-associated cancers, the only other cancer sites which have been discussed in relation to dietary fat or cholesterol are stomach cancer and lung cancer.

The trends in stomach cancer incidence and mortality are sharply declining in most countries and frequently in an inverse relation to colon cancer. Therefore, putative risk factors for colon cancer have frequently been considered protective for stomach cancer. This role has been assigned to dietary fat, among others, [58] but the epidemiological evidence supporting this is limited [59].

As far as lung cancer is concerned, two correlation studies [60,61] demonstrate an association between lung cancer mortality and per capita consumption of dietary fat. The more recent study [61] attempts to adjust for consumption data for tobacco. A case-control study on lung cancer in Hawaii [62] showed in males a significant association of lung cancer risk with dietary cholesterol intake after adjustment for other major risk factors and potential confounders. A similar relationship for females was not found.

A Canadian case-control study on bladder cancer also found an increased risk associated with dietary cholesterol intake [63].

Discussion

Critical assessment of the role of dietary fat and/or cholesterol intake in the aetiology of colorectal cancer and kidney cancer obviously has to deal with the methodological issues of properly assessing intake of these nutrients in populations studied [65]. While there seems to be a large variation of dietary fat intake between different populations which correlates strongly with the incidence or mortality of colorectal and/or kidney cancer, studies within populations could not identify such a large variation of dietary habits and an association of these with cancer risks. Only few of the studies mentioned above have used thoroughly evaluated methodologies in assessing dietary habits, while many used simple instruments, the validity of which had not been assessed. This can lead to a considerable degree of misclassification in the assessment of exposure and may have contributed to the problem of identifying clear-cut effects of dietary fat intake on cancer risk [65].

In addition, dietary habits represent a complex exposure with correlations between different foods and nutrients. Isolated analyses concerning single food items or nutrients need thoroughly to account for other factors. This is frequently not done to the extent necessary, so that effects of residual confounding cannot be excluded either. In quantitative terms these shortcomings can contribute to diminishing or disguising a true effect of dietary fat intake, but in the absence of solid data regarding the actual degree of misclassification [66] occurring when assessing dietary fat intake in epidemiological studies, it is difficult to estimate the size of this effect or even its existence.

In summary, the studies reviewed do not provide unequivocal evidence for a concrete role of dietary fat intake in the aetiology of colorectal and kidney cancer; however, the associations identified equally do not rule out a role of dietary fat since the risk factors identified in terms of foods, nutrients, dietary habits and their consequences are all to a considerable extent associated with high fat intake.

Acknowledgement

The secretarial assistance of Heike Neff is gratefully acknowledged.

REFERENCES

1 Committee on Diet, Nutrition, and Cancer: Diet, Nutrition, and Cancer. Washington DC: National Academy Press 1982

2 Armstrong BK, McMichael AJ, MacLennan R: Diet. In: Schottenfeld D and Fraumeni JF Jr (eds) Cancer Epidemiology and Prevention. Philadelphia: WB Saunders 1982:419-433

3 Joossens JV, Hill MJ, Geboers J (eds): Diet and Human Carcinogenesis. Amsterdam: Experta Medica 1985

4 Ip C, Birt DF, Rogers AE, Mettlin C (eds): Dietary Fat and Cancer. Progress in Clinical and Biological Research, Volume 222. New York: Alan R Liss Inc 1986

5 Graham S, Mettlin C: Diet and colon cancer. Am J Epidemiol 1979 (109):1-20

6 Zaridze DG: Environmental etiology of large-bowel cancer. J Natl Cancer Inst 1983 (70):389-400

7 Riboli E, Sasco AJ: Current hypothesis on the etiology of colorectal cancer. Critical review of the epidemiological evidence. Soz Praeventivmed 1986 (31):78-80

8 Trichopoulos D, Polychronopoulon A: Epidemiology, diet and colorectal cancer. Env J Cancer Clin Oncol 1986 (22):335-337

9 McMichael AJ, Jensen OM, Parkin DM, Zaridze DG: Dietary and endogenous cholesterol and human cancer. Epidemiol Reviews 1984 (6):192-216

10 Willett WC, MacMahon B: Diet and cancer - an overview. N Engl J Med 1984 (310):633-638 and 697-701

11 Kolonel LN, Le Marchand L: The epidemiology of colon cancer and dietary fat. In: Ip C, Birt DF, Rogers AE, Mettlin, C (eds) Dietary Fat and Cancer, Progress in Clinical and Biological Research, Volume 222

12 Drasar BS, Irving D: Environmental factors and cancer of the colon and breast. Br J Cancer 1973 (27):167-172

13 Armstrong B, Doll R: Environmental factors and cancer incidence and mortality in different countries with special reference to dietary practices. Int J Cancer 1975 (15):617-631

14 Knox EG: Foods and diseases. Br J Prev Soc Med 1977 (31):71-80

15 McKeown-Eyssen GE, Bright-See E: Dietary factors in colon cancer: International relationships. Nutr Cancer 1984 (6):160-170

16 Enstrom JE: Colorectal cancer and consumption of beef and fat. Br J Cancer 1975 (32):432-439

17 Bingham SA, Williams DRR, Cole TJ, James WPT: Dietary fibre and regional large-bowel cancer mortality in Britain. Br J Cancer 1979 (40):456-463

18 McMichael AJ, Potter JD, Hetzel BS: Time trends in colo-rectal cancer mortality in relation to food and alcohol consumption: United States, United Kingdom, Australia and New Zealand. Int J Epidemiol 1979 (8):295-303

19 Lyon JL, Sorenson W: Colon cancer in a low-risk population. Am J Clin Nutr 1978 (31):227-230

20 Kolonel LN, Hankin JH, Nomura AMY, Chu SY: Dietary fat intake and cancer incidence among five ethnic groups in Hawaii. Cancer Res 1981 (41):3727-3728.

21 Smith AH, Pearce NE, Joseph JG: Major colorectal cancer aetiological hypotheses do not explain mortality trends among Maori and non-Maori New Zealanders. Int J Epidemiol 1985 (14):79-85

22 Liu K, Moss D, Persky V, Stamler J, Garside D, Soltero I: Dietary cholesterol, fat, and fibre, and colon cancer mortality. An analysis of international data. Lancet 1979 (ii):782-785

23 International Agency for Research on Cancer Intestinal Microecology Group: Dietary fibre, transit time, faecal bacteria, steroids and colon cancer in two Scandinavian populations. Lancet 1977 (ii):207-211

24 Jensen OM, MacLennan R, Wahrendorf J (on behalf of the IARC large bowel cancer group): Diet, bowel function, fecal characteristics, and large bowel cancer in Denmark and Finland. Nutr Cancer 1982 (4):5-19

25 Reddy BS, Wynder EL: Large-bowel carcinogenesis: Fecal constituents of populations with diverse incidence rates of colon cancer. J Natl Cancer Inst 1973 (50):1437-1442

26 Jain M, Cook GM, Davis FG, Grace MG, Howe GR, Miller AB: A case-control study of diet and colo-rectal cancer. Int J Cancer 1980 (26):757-768

27 Miller AB, Howe GR, Jain M, Craib KJP, Harrison L: Food items and food groups as risk factors in a case-control study of diet and colo-rectal cancer. Int J Cancer 1983 (32):155-161

28 Wynder EL, Kajitani T, Ishikawa S, Dodo H, Takano A: Environmental factors of cancer of the colon and rectum. II.Japanese Epidemiological Data. Cancer 1969 (23):1210-1220

29 Dales LG, Friedman GD, Ury HK, Grossman, S, Williams SR: A case-control study of relationships of diet and other traits to colorectal cancer in American Blacks. Am J Epidemiol 1979 (109):132-144

30 Pickle LW, Greene MH, Ziegler RG, Toledo A, Hoover R, Lynch HT, Fraumeni JF: Colorectal cancer in rural Nebraska. Cancer Res 1984 (44):363-369

31 Modan B, Barell V, Lubin F, Modan M, Greenberg RA, Graham S: Low-fiber intake as an etiological factor in cancer of the colon. J Natl Cancer Inst 1975 (55):15-18

32 Wynder, EL, Shigematsu T: Environmental factors and cancer of the colon and rectum. Cancer 1967 (20):1520-1561

33 Manousos O, Day NE, Trichopoulos D, Gerovassilis F, Tzonou A, Polychronopoulou A: Diet and colorectal cancer: a case-control study in Greece. Int J Cancer 1983 (32):1-5

34 Haenszel W, Berg JW, Segi M, Kurihara M, Locke FB: Large bowel cancer in Hawaiian Japanese. J Natl Cancer Inst 1973 (51):1765-1779

35 Kune S, Kune GA, Watson LF: Case-control study of dietary etiological factors: The Melbourne Colorectal Cancer Study. Nutr Cancer 1987 (9):21-42.
36 Macquart-Moulin G, Riboli E, Cornée J, Charnay B, Berthezène P, Day N: Case-control study on colorectal cancer and diet in Marseille. Int J Cancer 1986 (38):183-191.
37 Potter JD, McMichael AJ: Diet and cancer of the colon and rectum: A case-control study. J Natl Cancer Inst 1986 (76):557-569.
38 Lyon JL, Mahoney AW, West DW, Gardner JW, Smith KR, Sorenson AW, Stanish W: Energy intake: Its relationship to colon cancer risk. J Natl Cancer Inst 1987 (78):853-861.
39 Tuyns AJ, Haelterman M, Kaaks R: Colorectal cancer and the intake of nutrients: Oligosaccharides are a risk factor, fats are not. A case-control study in Belgium. Nutr Cancer 1987 (10):181-196.
40 Esser W, Weithofer G, Bloch R: Zur Bedeutung des Fett- und Rohfasergehalts der Nahrung für die Entstehung des Kolonkarzinoms. Z.Gastroenterologie 1980 (18):30-37.
41 Hoff G, Moen IE, Trygg K, Frolich W, Sauar J, Vatn M: Epidemiology of polyps in the rectum and sigmoid colon. Scand J Gastroenterol 1986 (21):199-204.
42 Macquart-Moulin G, Riboli E, Cornée J, Kaaks R, Berthezène P: Colorectal polyps and diet: A case-control study in Marseille. Int J Cancer 1987 (40):179-188.
43 Willett WC, Sampson L, Stampfer MJ, Rosner B, Bain C, Witschi J, Hennekens CH, Speizer FE: Reproducibility and validity of a semiquantitative food frequency questionnaire. Am J Epidemiol 1985 (122):51-65
44 Block G, Hartman AM, Dresser CM, Carrol MD, Gannon J, Gardner L: A data-based approach to diet questionnaire design and testing. Am J Epidemiol 1986 (124):453-469
45 Stemmermann GN, Nomura AMY, Heilbrun LK: Dietary fat and the risk of colorectal cancer. Cancer Res 1984 (44):4633-37
46 Hirayama T: A large-scale cohort study on the relationship between diet and selected cancers of digestive organs. In: Bruce WR, Correa P, Lipkin M, Tannenbaum SR, Wilkins TD (eds.) Banbury Report 7: Gastrointestinal Cancer: Endogenous Factors. Cold Spring Harbor, NY: Cold Spring Harbor Laboratory 1981 pp 409-429
47 Garland C, Shekelle RB, Barrett-Connor E, Criqui MH, Rossof AH, Paul O: Dietary vitamin D and calcium and risk of colorectal cancer: A 19-year prospective study in men. Lancet 1985 (i):307-309
48 Phillips RL, Snowdon DA: Dietary relationships with fatal colorectal cancer among Seventh-Day Adventistis. J Natl Cancer Inst 1985 (74):307-317
49 Stampfer MJ, Willett WC, Colditz GA, Rosner B, Hennekens C, Speizer FE: A prospective study of diet and colon cancer in a cohort of women. Fed Proc 1987 (46): 883
50 Lew EA, Garfinkel L: Variations in mortality by weight among 750,000 men and women. J Chron Dis 1979 (32):563-576.
51 Wynder EL, Mabuchi K, Whitmore WF Jr: Epidemiology of adenocarcinoma of the kidney. J Natl Cancer Inst 1974 (53):1619-1634
52 Yu MC, Mack TM, Hanisch R, Cicioni C, Henderson BE: Cigarette smoking, obesity, diuretic use, and coffee consumption as risk factors for renal cell carcinoma. J Natl Cancer Inst 1986 (77):351-356
53 Goodman MT, Morgenstern H, Wynder EL: A case-control study of factors affecting the development of renal cell cancer. Am J Epidemiol 1986 (124):926-940
54 McLaughlin JK, Mandel JS, Blot WJ, Schuman LM, Mehl ES, Fraumeni JF: A population-based case-control study of renal cell carcinoma. J Natl Cancer Inst 1984 (72):275-284
55 Maclure KM, MacMahon B: Dietary protein, obesity and other risk factors for renal adenocarcinoma. 1988 (submitted for publication)
56 Armstrong B, Garrod A, Doll R: A retrospective study of renal cancer with special reference to coffee and animal protein consumption. Br J Cancer 1976 (33):127-136
57 McCredie M, Ford JM, Stewart JH: Risk factors for cancer of the renal parenchyma. 1988 (submitted for publication)
58 Hill MJ: Dietary fat and human cancer (review). Anticancer Res 1987 (7):281-292
59 Kinlen LJ, Hermon C, Smith PG: A proportionate study of cancer mortality among members of a vegetarian society. Br J Cancer 1983 (48):355-361
60 Carroll KK, Khor HT: Dietary fat in relation to tumorigenesis. Prog Biochem Pharmacol 1975 (10):308-353
61 Wynder EL, Hebert JR, Kabat GC: Association of dietary fat and lung cancer. J Natl Cancer Inst 1987 (79):631-637
62 Hinds MW, Kolonel LN, Hankin LN, Lee J: Dietary cholesterol and lung cancer risk in a multiethnic population in Hawaii. Int J Cancer 1983 (32):727-732
63 Risch HA, Burch JD, Miller AB, Hill GB, Steele R and Howe GR: Dietary factors and the incidence of cancer of the urinary bladder. Am J Epidemiol 1988 (in press)
64 Mettlin C: Methodological issues in epidemiologic studies of dietary fat and cancer. In: Ip C. Birt DF, Rogers AE, Mettlin C (eds) Dietary Fat and Cancer, Progress in Clinical and Biological Research, Volume 222. 1986:3-15
65 Wahrendorf J: Questionnaire-derived historic dietary information. In: Joossens JV, Hill MJ and Geboers J (eds) Diet and Human Carcinogenesis. Amsterdam: Experta Medica 1985: 245-252
66 Blettner M, Wahrendorf J: What does an observed relative risk convey about possible misclassification? Meth Inf Med 1984 (23):37-40

Dietary Fibre Carbohydrate and Cancer: Epidemiologic Evidence

Ole M. Jensen

Danish Cancer Registry, Institute of Cancer Epidemiology of the Danish Cancer Society, Landskronagade 66, DK-2100 Copenhagen, Denmark

Introduction

The removal of "roughage" from food has led to an increasingly refined and calorie-dense diet in the economically developed parts of the world. In the early 1970s, it was suggested that this low-fibre diet was responsible for the high risk of large bowel cancer in the westernized parts of the world, and also to play a role for a number of other diseases characteristic of Western societies such as appendicitis, diverticulosis, hemorrhoids and varicose veins [1].

This suggested protection by fibre has stimulated not only experimental and epidemiological research on large bowel cancer, but also studies into the physiological properties of dietary fibre. Although this has revealed an increasingly complex situation, a protective effect of fibre is biologically plausible. However, epidemiological evidence of the protection by fibre has mainly been based on observation of differences in colon cancer incidence between populations and on the results of ecological studies. Such evidence is normally regarded as rather weak, and when the US National Academy of Science reviewed the role of Diet, Nutrition and Cancer in 1981 [2], no conclusive evidence was found "to indicate that dietary fibre (such as that present in certain fruits, vegetables, grains and cereals) exerts a protective effect against colorectal cancer and humans". In a more recent review, Willett and MacMahon [3] concluded that "although the available epidemiologic data are not entirely consistent, the weight of the evidence generally supports the hypothesis that fibre protects against colon cancer", and Greenwald et al. [4] in their evaluation found clear suggestions of "a relationship between colon cancer and diet low in fibre".

Early case-control studies in the 1970s looked at the association between colorectal cancer and fibre-rich foods. By contrast several case-control studies have been conducted during the 1980s on diet and colorectal cancer to test the hypothesis of a protective role of dietary fibre against these tumours. The main emphasis of this review will be placed on the results emerging from such studies of individuals focusing on dietary fibre rather than fibre-rich foods.

Biological Effects of Dietary Fibre

The fraction of food resistant to acids and alkaline (i.e., crude fibre) bears little relation to the physiologically active fibres defined as "skeletal remains of plant cells that are resistant to digestion by enzymes of man" [5]. Dietary fibre is measured today as the non-starch polysaccharides (NSP) which are quantitatively the major components of plant cell walls [6]. The main components are cellulose, hemicellulose, pectin, gums and the "noncarbohydrate" lignin.

Burkitt [1] proposed that dietary fibre protects against colorectal cancer by increasing faecal bulk, reducing mouth-anus transit time and possibly changing the bacterial flora of the gut. Indeed, dietary fibre increases the volume i.e. stool weight, since the fibres have water binding capacities and, in addition, they provide a substrate for bacterial proliferation which also leads to large stools. The dilution of a constant amount of cancer promoting substance, e.g. secondary bile acids, in a larger volume leads to a lowering of the concentration in the lumen of the gut.

Other properties of dietary fibre may also modify cancer risk. The fermentation of pectin, hemicellulose and gum lead to the production of short-chain fatty acids, among which butyrate may be an important intermediate in colonic mucosal metabolism, influencing cell differentiation [7]. Fermentation may stimulate bacterial growth, and it leads to a lowering of the pH in the gut, which influences enzymatic activity. At high pH (i.e., low fibre) this may lead to an increased degradation of bile acids to secondary bile acids. Bile acids are absorbed by dietary fibre. A reduction in the concentration of free ammonium (NH_4^+) and a lowering of serum cholesterol by removal of bile acids from the entero-hepatic circulation are additional properties of dietary fibres.

Dietary fibre thus influences bowel physiology in several complex ways, and the different components of total dietary fibre have different biological effects. The epidemiologist is faced with the problems provided by these incompletely understood biological properties when he attempts to understand the association between cancer and dietary fibre, most often measured by crude methods in their totality, and often without any possibility of distinguishing the consumption of individual fibre fractions.

Colorectal Cancer

Ecological Studies

As reviewed previously [8,9], cancer of the large bowel is a disease of affluent, westernized cultures of Europe, North America, Australia and New Zealand. The low incidence and mortality rates in Japan point to Western life-style rather than industrialization as being of importance. This is underscored by the increase in colorectal cancer incidence observed when Japanese migrate to the United States [10].

In most of the high-risk countries, large bowel cancer ranks among the 5 leading sites of cancer [9,10], and when considered together cancer of these sites represent one of the most prominent cancer problems in countries with westernized life-styles.

When Drasar and Irving [11] correlated national consumption levels of crude fibre with mortality rates of colon or rectum cancer, no association was found; when a correlation emerged in the study by Liu et al. [12], it was secondary to cholesterol intake. However, a weak inverse international correlation emerged from a recent analysis, where national colon cancer mortality rates were compared with the availability of dietary fibre defined as non-starch polysaccharides, and adjustment was undertaken for consumption of meats and fats [13,14].

In Britain, Bingham et al. [15] in 1979 described a non-significant inverse correlation between dietary fibre intake and regional death rates from colon cancer. A highly significant protective effect of pentosans was described. However, this could not be confirmed in a renewed analysis [16] where fibre intake was redefined as non-starch polysaccharides. By contrast, a significant inverse association was found for total dietary fibre, but it should be noted that the association was found within a very narrow range from 11.8-13.2 g dietary fibre per day over the various regions, as illustrated in Fig. 1.

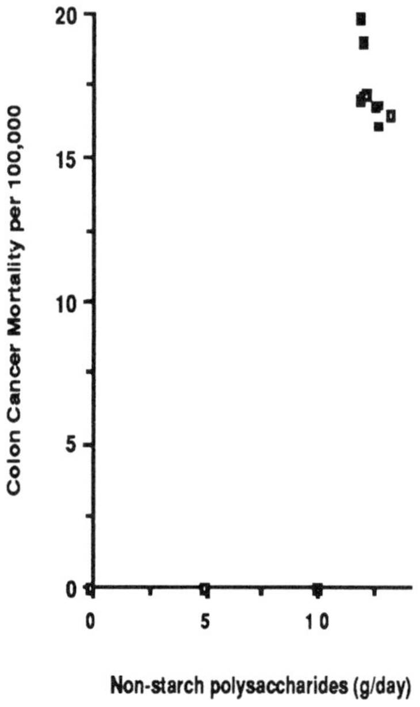

Fig. 1. Regional dietary fibre consumption (non-starch polysaccharides, g/day) in relation to colon cancer mortality (truncated (35-64 year) age-standardized rates) in England and Wales. r= -0.72.
(After: Bingham et al. [16])

Table 1. Colon cancer incidence and daily intake of dietary fib... d. Males. (Source: Jensen et al. [18])

	Finland rural	Denma... rural		
Colon cancer incidence/100,000	6.7	12.9		
Colorectal cancer incidence /100,000	14.2	27.9		
Fat (g/day)	133	146		
Total fibre (g/day) [a]	18.4	18.0	1[illegible]	
Pentose (g/day)	7.4	6.6	5.5	
Hexose (g/day)	5.3	5.5	3.7	
Uronic acid (g/day)	1.9	2.2	2.0	
Cellulose (g/day)	4.1	3.7	3.4	[illegible].2

a) Significant inverse trend with large bowel cancer

The most careful studies which contrast fibre consumption in populations with differences in colorectal cancer incidence have been coordinated by the International Agency for Research on Cancer [17,18], In the second study [18], fibre intake was determined as non-starch polysaccha-rides by chemical analysis of duplicate portions [19] eaten by random samples of men in Finland and Denmark. Total dietary fibre intake was significantly higher in the low-risk Finnish population than in Denmark, both groups having similar daily fat intakes (Table 1).

The dietary fibre intake was also higher in North Sweden than in New York City, where the risk of colon cancer is high [20]. In the United States the low risk Seventh Day Adventists had a higher intake of dietary fibre than the general US population [21], while no difference in fibre intake was seen for the Maori and the non-Maori groups of the New Zealand population [22], in spite of the fact that the non-Maoris have a 2-3 times higher colon cancer incidence than the Maoris [10]. Similarly, no difference in daily fibre consumption was seen for population groups in South Africa with variation in colon cancer incidence [23]. In Japan, a low incidence country for colorectal cancer [10], the intake of dietary fibre measured as non-starch polysaccharides was as low as in the 1950s, 1960s and 1970s as in high risk Copenhagen and Britain [24]; no secular trend in fibre consumption was noted in Japan where colon cancer incidence and mortality have increased rapidly.

In addition to such studies of fibre intake and colon cancer, several national and international investigations have compared the consumption of high-fibre foods (cereals, vegetables, fruits) for populations with differences in colorectal cancer incidence. Inverse correlations have almost invariably been found with cereals [25-28], but this did not persist in one study where account was taken of the possible influence of other dietary factors such as meats and fats [26], which were associated with an increased colorectal cancer risk. A positive correlation was found with sugar intake in that same study. In Hong Kong, fibre-rich foods and vegetables were taken in larger amounts by the high-risk than by the low-risk socioeconomic groups [29], but so were all other foods. In low-risk rural Finland, cereal consumption was high compared with high-risk New York [30] and Copenhagen [31].

Studies of Individuals

In contrast to the ecological studies based on group comparisons, case-control and cohort studies assess the consumption of dietary

Table 2. Summary of the association between dietary fibre consumption and colorectal cancer risk in case-control studies

Study area, year (Ref.)	No. of cases, controls	Source of controls	Method of dietary assessment	Summary of results
Israel 1975 [34]	275, 510 (colon: 198) (rectum: 77)	Hospital Neighbourhood	Food frequency	Decreased risk of colon cancer among consumers of high-fibre foods Rectal cancer not associated with fibre
Norway/USA 1978 [35]	Norway: 278, 1394 (colon: 162) (rectum: 116) Minnesota: 373, 1657 (colon: 259) (rectum: 114)	Hospital	Food frequency	Decreased risk of colorectal cancer among fibre consumers
USA 1978 [36]	99,280	Hospital and multiphasic health checkup	Food frequency	Non-significant decreased risk of colon cancer among high fibre consumers
Puerto Rico 1979 [37]	461, 461	Community	Food frequency	Increased risk of colorectal cancer associated with high fibre consumption
Germany FR 1980 [38]	49, 60 (colon: ?: 49; incl. 30 adenomas)	Hospital	Food diary	Mean intake of crude fibre identical for cases and controls
Canada 1980, 1983, 1986 [39,40,41]	542, 1077 (colon: 348) (rectum: 194)	Hospital Neighbourhood	Diet history	No association with consumption of crude fibre for colon or rectum cancer
France 1986 [42]	399,399	Hospital	Diet history	Significant decrease in colorectal cancer risk with increasing consumption of fibre in vegetables. Association disappeared after adjustment for other nutrient differences
Australia 1986 [44]	419, 732 (colon: 220) (rectum: 199)	Population-based	Self-administered quantitative food frequency	Increasing risk of colorectal cancer associated with fibre intake, in particular cereal fibre
Australia 1987 [45]	715, 727 (colon: 392) (rectum: 323)	Community (interviewed separately from cases)	Diet history	Decreased risk of colorectal cancer associated with high fibre intake from any source. No adjustments for other dietary factors
USA 1987 [46]	246, 484 (colon: 246)	Community	Diet history	Weak inconsistent decreased risk of colon cancer with increasing fibre consumption after adjustment for total energy intake
Belgium 1987 [47]	1235, 3524 (colon: 704) (rectum: 531)	Community	Diet history	Significant decreased risk of colon and rectum cancer with increasing fibre consumption after adjustment for total energy intake

fibres as well as exposure to other potential risk factors in individuals who have developed or may develop colorectal cancer.

The intake of dietary fibre has not been reported in cohort studies in relation to colorectal cancer development. In Hirayama's prospective cohort study [32], the higher the daily intake of rice and wheat, the lower the standardized mortality ratio for colon and rectal cancer. These foods supposedly provide the greater amount of dietary fibre in Japan [33].

The results of case-control studies which attempt to examine the influence of dietary fibre on colon or colorectal cancer are summarized in Table 2. The estimates of fibre intake in these studies range from the consumption of fibre foods taken as proxy measures for fibre intake over food table based crude fibre intake to dietary fibre intakes defined as non-starch polysaccharides. Few studies have attempted to relate colorectal cancer risk to different fibre components. The results of the studies of individuals are highly conflicting, ranging from significant protective effects over no association with dietary fibre intake to an increasing risk of colorectal cancer with fibre consumption.

Early studies were carried out in the 1970s. In 1975 Modan et al. [34] reported that the consumption of high-fibre foods was lower among colon cancer cases in Israel than among controls, while no difference was seen for rectal cancer. In Norway and the United States (Minnesota) a decreased risk of colorectal cancer was associated with a somewhat higher consumption of crude fibre [35], but neither the relative risk nor the fibre consumption were given by the author. In California, Dales et al. [36] compared the diets of black colorectal cancer patients and controls selected from hospitals and a multiphasic health check-up programme. The study had a very low participation rate of around 40-50%. A non-significant decreased risk was seen among consumers of fibre-rich foods, in particular for colon cancer. A significantly increased relative risk was seen for consumers of high fat/low fibre diets. By contrast, the risk of colorectal cancer increased with increasing consumption of fibre-rich foods in a large population-based case-control study in Puerto Rico [37], but the diets of some 25% of the study subjects were assessed by proxy interviews with relatives. In a small hospital study in the Federal Republic of Germany, the mean intake of crude fibre was identical for patients with and without colon cancer or polyps [38]. No adjustments were made for total calorie intake in any of these studies.

A large case-control study was conducted in 3 provinces of Canada, and dietary information from cases of colon cancer and rectum cancer was compared with that of population and hospital controls. No protective effect was found in the initial analysis of crude fibre [39] or in the later assessment of the influence of total dietary fibre on colon or rectum cancer risk [40]. The possible confounding effect of other risk factors for colorectal cancer was controlled, and in a reanalysis of the association of colorectal cancer with crude dietary fibre intake [41] the Authors concluded that there was no evidence for any protective effect of fibre even after adjustment for total calorie intake.

In a large hospital-based study in the south of France [42] there was a significant decrease in colorectal cancer risk for increasing consumption of vegetables with a low and medium fibre content, but this association faded when an adjustment was made for other dietary factors. No analysis was performed for total dietary fibre consumption, and the possible effects of fibre and other components of vegetables cannot be distinguished. No association was seen between colorectal cancer and the consumption of monosaccharides. In a parallel study [43] of patients with colorectal polyps and hospital controls no protective effect was discernible for total dietary fibre, although the relative risk decreased with increasing intake of fibres from fruits, vegetables and potatoes. A protective effect was seen in that study for carbohydrate consumption minus added sugars.

Two studies in Australia have provided opposite results. Potter and McMichael [44] in 1986 reported on a large population-based study of colorectal cancer where dietary information was obtained by means of a validated self-administered quantitative food frequency questionnaire. On the contrary, the risk of colorectal cancer increased with increasing total fibre consumption. This was highly significant in women and the association was not influenced by adjustment for total calorie intake. In Melbourne, Kune et al. [45] recorded the diet histories of colorectal cancer patients and subsequently they recorded similar information from age and sex-matched controls selected from the population at large. The risk of colorectal cancer decreased significantly with total fibre consumption and with the consumption of foods providing dietary fibre. The strongest protective effect was found for a diet with a high fibre content and a high vegetable component. However, there seemed to be no dose-effect relationship, and the associations reported were not adjusted for the possible influence of other dietary factors.

In the United States (Utah), Lyon et al. [46] conducted a population-based study of colon cancer focusing a diet history on eating habits 5 years prior to interview. A slight increase in the risk for colon cancer associated with crude fibre intake was reversed to a weak, inconsistent protective effect when the risk estimates were adjusted for total energy intake. The association was more evident in women than in men, but no information on statistical significance was provided.

In Belgium, Tuyns et al. [47] studied 1235 large bowel cancer patients (704 colon cancer; 531 rectal cancer) and 3524 controls drawn from the general population. Information on food consumption was obtained by means of a diet history questionnaire similar to the one used in the Marseille study. Significant decreasing relative risks of both colon and rectal cancer were seen to be associated with increasing consumption of dietary fibre also after adjustment for total caloric intake. Increasing relative risk of both colon and rectum cancer were also seen for the consumption of oligosaccharides. A similar finding was described by Bristol et al. [48] from the United Kingdom, where no association emerged for dietary fibre.

Several further case-control studies have shown a protective effect of vegetable consumption against colorectal cancer in widely different countries as the United States [49], Japan [50] and Greece [51].

Cancers of Other Sites

Hakama and Saxen [52] found a strong correlation with the per capita intake of cereal used as flour and mortality for *stomach cancer*. In a further evaluation of the possible association between carbohydrate intake and cancer, Modan et al. [53] found that high-starch foods were consumed more frequently by cases than by controls in Israel. Similarly, in a case-control study of diet and stomach cancer in Canada [54], a trend of increasing risk with consumption of carbohydrate as a whole was found. Increasing consumption of dietary fibre was associated with a significant decreasing risk of stomach cancer in that study.

Adlercreutz [55] speculated that a fibre-rich diet may influence estrogen metabolism by inhibiting reabsorption of biliary estrogens and that plant lignans may serve as precursors for animal lignans with hormonal or antihormonal effects. He suggested that fibre in the diet may be the linking factor for the association between colon and *breast cancer* incidence in whole populations [9] and in individuals [56,57]. The possible role of fibre was supported by the observation of associations between fibre intake and lignans and various sex hormones in women [58,59]. In a large case-control study in Israel, Lubin et al. [60] employed a food frequency questionnaire. They found a decreasing risk with the increasing consumption of fibre-containing foods among younger, but not among older women. Total fibre consumption was not evaluated. By contrast, no association was found with wholemeal bread or pasta in an Italian case-control study [62].

Further positive correlations were reported by Armstrong and Doll [26] between sugar intake and cancer of the colon, rectum, breast, ovary, prostate, kidney, nervous system and testicles; there was an inverse correlation for incidence of liver cancer.

Comments and Conclusions

The current epidemiologic evidence is insufficient to conclude that the consumption of dietary fibre offers protection against colorectal cancer - the only cancer in which the possible association has been investigated in detail in a large number of studies. Inconsistent results have emerged from the ecological studies, but the definition of fibre has not always been optimal. When the correlations observed were controlled for the consumption of fats and meats, a weak, inconsistent, inverse relation with fibre consumption remained only in one study. The best indication of a high cereal fibre intake has emerged from the observation of a high cereal fibre intake in low-risk Finland compared with high-incidence populations of Denmark and the United States. However, these results have not been corroborated in other populations showing similar variations in colorectal cancer incidence. Even if ecologic studies cover a large variation in fibre consumption, the informative value of such studies is limited. In the studies of fibre, no account was thus taken of a possible temporal relation between exposure and cancer occurrence, and information on exposure and effect (i.e., consumption of dietary fibre and cancer mortality or incidence) has often been obtained from different population groups. Furthermore, a multitude of factors other than fibre consumption are likely to differ between the populations included in such studies without considering their possible influence on cancer risk.

Early case-control studies pointed to a protective role of fresh fruit and vegetables which are important sources of dietary fibre. Recent large and well-conducted studies have, with one or two exceptions, either shown no protective effect of dietary fibre or only weak and inconsistent associations with colorectal cancer, when fibre intake was measured by means of dietary questionnaires of various sorts.

The available results of case-control studies are insufficient to conclude that there is a true association between dietary fibre intake and colorectal cancer. Nor can such an association be rejected on the basis of currently available studies. A protective effect of dietary fibre may just not be detectable by current case-control methodology. Case-control studies are prone to bias, which may be particularly serious when studying the association between diet and large bowel cancer, since the disease itself may lead to dietary changes. The direction of such bias may be unpredictable. When measuring the protective effect of dietary fibre by case-control methodology, a further difficulty is related to misclassification resulting from measurement errors. This may be particularly important in populations with a low dietary fibre consumption and with limited variation in intake between individuals. All the more recent case-control studies have been conducted in populations with such characteristics. Misclassification is further enhanced, as the instruments for assessing food intake may be too crude. It is also difficult or impossible to take account of the temporal relationship between exposure (i.e., fibre consumption) and cancer occurrence in case-control studies, and difficulties arise if total dietary fibre is only a proxy measure for the truly biologically important factors such as, for instance, a given fibre fraction. The composite effect of misclassification is to bias relative risk estimates towards one - the no-effect level. Additional difficulties arise from the fact that several dietary factors are strongly intercorrelated and may have independent effects on colorectal cancer. In fact, several factors may jointly be responsible for colorectal cancer with dietary fibre playing a risk-modifying role against a background provided by other components of the diet.

With current methodological limitations for the study of diet, nutrition and cancer, the epidemiological findings must be seen together with the biological plausibility of the association, and with findings emerging from animal experiments. As reviewed elsewhere in this monograph [63], the experimental findings do not contribute substantially to a better understanding of the association. Observations in all fields encourage additional research, as the current uncertainty precludes firm recommendations on colorectal prevention by supplementation of the diet with dietary fibre. The indications of a lower risk of colorectal and other cancers in consumers of fresh fruit and vegetables justify, however, general dietary recommendations to increase the consumption of these food components, which are not known to be associated with undesirable side effects.

Acknowledgement

Ms Ulla Madsen assisted with the retrieval of literature, and Mrs Aase Falck with the preparation of the manuscript.

REFERENCES

1 Burkitt DP: Epidemiology of cancer of the colon and rectum. Cancer 1971 (28):3-13
2 National Research Council: Diet, Nutrition and Cancer. Washington DC: National Academy Press 1982:130-137
3 Willett WC and McMahon B: Diet and cancer - an overview. N Engl J Med 1984 (310):633-638, 697-703
4 Greenwald P, Lanza E, Eddy GA: Dietary fibre in the reduction of colon cancer risk. J Am Diet Ass 1987 (87):1178-1188
5 Trowell H, Burkitt D, Heaton K (eds) Dietary Fibre, Fibre-Depleted Foods and Disease. London: Academic Press 1985
6 Englyst H, Wiggins, HS, Cummings JH: Determination of the non-starch polysaccharides in plant foods by gas-liquid chromatography of constituent sugars as alditol acetates. Analyst 1982 (107):307-318
7 Roediger WEW: Role of aerobic bacteria in the metabolic welfare of the colonic mucosa in man. Gut 1980 (21):793-798
8 Jensen OM: Colon cancer epidemiology. In: Autrup H, Williams GM (eds) Experimental Colon Carcinogenesis. Boca Raton: CRC Press 1983:3-23
9 Boyle P, Zaridze DG, Smans M: Descriptive epidemiology of colorectal cancer. Int J Cancer 1985 (36):9-18
10 Waterhouse J, Muir C, Shanmugaratnam K, Powel K: Cancer Incidence in Five Continents. Vol IV. IARC Scientific Publications No. 42. Lyon, International Agency for Research on Cancer 1982
11 Drasar BS and Irving D: Environmental factors in cancer of the colon and breast. Br J Cancer 1973 (27):167-172
12 Liu K, Stamler J, Moss D, Garside D, Persky V and Soltero I: Dietary cholesterol, fat and fibre, and colon cancer mortality. Lancet 1975 (II):782-785
13 McKeown-Eyssen and Bright-See E: Dietary factors in colon cancer: International relationships. Nutr Cancer 1984 (6):160-170
14 McKeown-Eyssen and Bright-See E: Dietary factors in colon cancer: International relationships. An update. Nutr Cancer 1985 (7):251-253
15 Bingham S, Williams DRR, Cole TJ and James WPT: Dietary fibre and regional large bowel cancer mortality in Britain. Br J Cancer 1979 (40):456-463
16 Bingham SA, Williams DRR and Cummings JH: Dietary fibre consumption in Britain: New estimates and their relation to large bowel cancer mortality. Br J Cancer 1985 (52):399-402
17 International Agency for Research on Cancer Intestinal Microecology Group: Dietary fibre, transit time, fecal bacteria, steroids, and colon cancer in two Scandinavian populations. Lancet 1977 (II):207-211
18 Jensen OM, MacLennan R and Wahrendorf J: Diet, bowel function, fecal characteristics and large bowel cancer in Denmark and Finland. Nutr Cancer 1982 (4):5-19
19 Englyst HN, Bingham SA, Wiggins HS, Southgate DAT, Seppänen R, Helms P, Anderson V, Day KC, Choolun R, Collison E and Cummings JH: Nonstarch polysaccharide consumption in four Scandinavian populations. Nutr Cancer 1982 (4):50-60
20 Domellöf L, Darby L, Hanson D, Mathews L, Simi B and Reddy BS: Fecal sterols and bacterial beta-glucuronidase activity: A preliminary metabolic epidemiology study of healthy volunteers from Umea, Sweden, and Metropolitan New York. Nutr Cancer 1982 (4):120-127
21 Kurup PA, Jayakumari N, Indira M, Muraleedhara Kurup G, Vargheese T, Mathew A, Goodman GT, Calkins BM, Kessie G, Turjman N and Nair PP: Diet, nutrition intake and metabolism in populations at high and low risk for colon cancer. Composition, intake, and excretion of fiber constituents. Am J Clin Nutr 1984 (49):123-127
22 Smith AH, Pearce NE and Joseph JG: Major colorectal cancer aetiological hypotheses do not explain mortality trends among Maori and non-Maori New Zealanders. Int J Epidemiol 1985 (14):79-85
23 Walker ARP, Walker BF and Walker AJ: Faecal pH, dietary fibre intake, and proneness to colon cancer in four South African populations. Br J Cancer 1986 (53):489-495
24 Kuratsune M, Honda T, Englyst HN and Cummings JH: Dietary fiber in the Japanese diet as investigated in connection with colon cancer risk. Jpn J Cancer Res (Gann) 1986 (77):736-738
25 Irving D and Drasar BS: Fiber and cancer of the colon. Br J Cancer 1973 (28):462-463
26 Armstrong B and Doll R: Environmental factors in cancer incidence and mortality in different countries, with special reference to dietary practices. Int J Cancer 1975 (15):617-631
27 Howell MA: Diet as an etiological factor in the development of cancers of the colon and rectum. J Chron Dis 1975 (28):67-80
28 Knox EG: Foods and diseases. Br J Prev Soc Med 1977 (31):71-80
29 Hill M, MacLennan R and Newcombe K: Diet and large bowel cancer in three socioeconomic groups in Hong Kong. Lancet 1979 (I):436
30 Reddy BS, Hedges A, Laakso K and Wynder EL: Fecal constituents of a high risk North American and a low risk Finnish population for the development of large bowel cancer. Cancer Letters 1978 (4):217-222
31 MacLennan R, Jensen OM, Mosbech J and Vuori H: Diet, transit time, stool weight and colon cancer in two Scandinavian populations. Am J Clin Nutr 1978 (31):239-242
32 Hirayama T: A large scale cohort study on the relationship between diet and selected cancer of digestive organs. In: Bruce WR, Correa P, Lipkin M, Tannenbaum SR, Wilkins TD (eds) Banbury Report 7. Gastrointestinal Cancer: Endogenous Factors. Cold Spring Harbor, N.Y.: Cold Spring Harbor Laboratory 1981:409-429
33 Zaridze DG: Environmental etiology of large bowel cancer. JNCI 1983 (70):389-400
34 Modan B, Barell V, Lubin F, Modan M, Greenberg RA and Graham S: Low fiber intake as an etiologic factor in cancer of the colon. JNCI 1975 (55):15-18
35 Bjelke E: Epidemiologic studies of cancer of the stomach, colon and rectum with special emphasis on the role of diet. Scand J Gastroenterol 1974 (9; Supplementum 31):1-235

36 Dales LG, Friedman GD, Ury HK, Grossman S and Williams SR: A case-control study of relationships of diet and other traits to colorectal cancer in American Blacks. Am J Epidemiol 1979 (199):132-144
37 Martinez I, Torres R, Frias Z, Colon JR and Fernandez N: Factors associated with adenocarcinomas of the large bowel in Puerto Rico. In: Advances in Medical Oncology, Research and Education, Vol 3. Oxford: Pergamon 1979:45-52
38 Esser W, Weithofer G and Bloch R: Zur Bedeutung des Fett- und Rohfasergehalts der Nahrung für die Entstehung des Kolonkarzinoms. Z Gasteroenterologie 1980 (18):1-8
39 Jain M, Cook GM, Davis FG, Grace MG, Howe GR and Miller AB: A case-control study of diet and colorectal cancer. Int J Cancer 1980 (26):757-768
40 Miller AB, Howe GR, Jain M, Craib KJP and Harrison L: Food items and food groups as risk factors in a case control study of diet and colorectal cancer. Int J Cancer 1983 (32):155-161
41 Howe GR, Miller AB and Jain M: Total energy intake: Implications for epidemiologic analyses. Am J Epidemiol 1986 (124):157-159
42 Macquart-Moulin G, Riboli E, Cornee J, Charnay B, Berthezene P and Day N: Case-control study on colorectal cancer and diet in Marseilles. Int J Cancer 1986 (38):183-191
43 Macquart-Moulin G, Riboli E, Cornee J, Kaaks R and Berthezene P: Colorectal polyps and diet: A case-control study in Marseilles. Int J Cancer 1987 (49):179-188
44 Potter JD and McMichael AJ: Diet and cancer of the colon and rectum: A case-control study. JNCI 1986 (76):557-569
45 Kune S, Kune GA and Watson LF: Case-control study of dietary etiological factors: The Melbourne colorectal cancer study. Nutr Cancer 1987 (9):21-42
46 Lyon JL, Mahoney AW, West DW, Gardner JW, Smith KR, Sorenson AW and Stanish W: Energy intake: Its relationship to colon cancer risk. JNCI 1987 (78):853-861
47 Tuyns AJ, Haelterman M and Kaaks R: Colorectal cancer and the intake of nutrients: Oligosaccharides are a risk factor, fats are not. A case-control study in Belgium. Nutr Cancer 1987 (10):181-196
48 Bristol JB, Emmot, Heaton KW and Williamson RC: Sugar, fat and the risk of colorectal cancer. Br Med J 1985 (291):1467-1470
49 Graham S, Dayal H, Swanson M, Mittelman A and Wilkinson G: Diet in the epidemiology of cancer of the colon and rectum. JNCI 1978 (61)709-714
50 Haenszel W, Locke FB and Segi M: A case-control study of large bowel cancer in Japan. JNCI 1980 (64):17-22
51 Manousos O, Day NE, Trichopoulos D, Gerovassilis F, Tzonou A and Polychronopoulou A: Diet and colorectal cancer: A case-control study in Greece. Int J Cancer 1983 (32):1-5
52 Hakama M and Saxen EA: Cereal consumption and gastric cancer. Int J Cancer 1967 (2):265-268
53 Modan BW, Lubin F, Barell V, Greenberg RA, Modan M and Graham S: The role of starches in the etiology of gastric cancer. Cancer 1974 (34):2087-2092
54 Rish HA, Jain M, Choi NW, Fodor JG, Pfeiffer CJ, Howe GR, Harrison LW, Czaib KJP and Miller AB: Dietary factors and the incidence of cancer of the stomach. Am J Epidemiol 1985 (122):947-957
55 Adlerkreutz H: Dose fiber-rich food containing animal lignan precursors protect against both colon and breast cancer? An extension of the "Fiber Hypothesis". Gastroenterol 1984 (86)761-766
56 Curtis RE, Boice JD, Kleinerman RA, Flannary JT and Fraumeni JF: Summary: Multiple primary cancers in Connecticut 1935-82. Natl Cancer Inst Monogr 1985 (68):219-242
57 Storm HH, Jensen OM, Ewertz M, Lynge E, Olsen JH, Schou G and Østerlind A: Summary: Multiple primary cancers in Denmark, 1943-80. Natl Cancer Inst Monogr 1985 (68):411-430
58 Adlercreutz H, Fotsis T, Heikkinen R, Dwyer JT, Woods M, Goldin BR, Gorbach SL: Excretion of the lignans enterolactone and enterodiol and of equol in onmivorous and vegetarian postmenopausal women and in women with breast cancer. Lancet 1982 (II):1295-1299
59 Adlercreutz H, Hökerstedt K, Bannwart C, Bloiger S, Hämäläinen E, Fotsis T and Ollus A: Effect of dietary components, including lignans and phytoestrogens on enterohepatic circulation and liver metabolism of estrogens and sex hormone binding globulin (SHBG). J Steroid Biochem 1987 (27):1135-1144
60 Lubin F, Wax Y and Modan B: Role of fat, animal protein and dietary fiber in breast cancer etiology: A case-control study. JNCI 1986 (77):605-611
61 La Vecchia C, Decarli A, Franceschi S, Gentile A, Negri E and Panazzini F: Dietary factors and the risk of breast cancer. Nutr Cancer 1987 (10):205-214
62 La Vecchia C, Decarli A, Fasoli M and Gentile A: Nutrition and diet in the etiology of endometrial cancer. Cancer 1986 (57):1248-1253
63 Hill MJ: Experimental studies of fat and fibre in carcinogenesis (present volume European School of Oncology Monographs)

Experimental Studies of Fat, Fibre and Calories in Carcinogenesis

M. J. Hill

PHLS-CAMR, Porton Down, Salisbury, Wilts SP4 OJG, United Kingdom

Introduction

Experimental studies of fat, fibre and calories have been concentrated on cancer of the large bowel and on cancer of the breast. Good models are available for the study of aspects of both cancers, but there is some controversy regarding their value in determining the role of diet in the causation of these cancers. This is especially so in colorectal carcinogenesis where the effect of dietary factors varies with the carcinogen and the strain of animal used.

Colorectal Cancer

Before reviewing the results of experimental studies of dietary fat and fibre it is first necessary to discuss the animal models used.

The animal models were reviewed recently [1,2] and the following is a summary. A wide variety of chemical carcinogens may be used, including aflatoxin, dimethylaminobiphenyl (DMAB), cycasin, dimethylhydrazine (DMH), azoxymethane (AOM), methylnitrosourea (MNU) and N-methyl-N-nitroso-N-nitrosoguanidine (MNNG). The latter two are direct acting carcinogens and must therefore be delivered intrarectally. Cycasin, methylazoxy-methanol-beta-glucoside, is given orally and is activated to the locally acting carcinogen methylazoxymethanol (MAM) by the action of bacterial beta-glucosidase in the animal gut. The most widely used carcinogens are AOM or DMH, both of which can be given subcutaneously. In the commonest model DMH is given in weekly subcutaneous injections of 15 mg/Kg; higher doses give acute toxicity whilst smaller doses give fewer tumours. AOM is administered at a dosage of 8 mg/Kg, and Table 1 gives the dose-response relationship for the production of intestinal tumours by AOM in rats.

Table 1. The dose-response relationship between subcutaneous AOM and intestinal tumour formation in male Sprague-Dawley rats

AOM Administration			Number of intestinal tumours per rat	
Dose (mg/Kg)	Number of weekly doses	% of rats with tumours	Small bowel	Large bowel
20	1	25	0.3	0.06
20	2	94	1.5	2.0
16	2	93	1.0	1.3
12	2	75	1.1	0.6
8	2	53	0.2	0.7
8	8	100	1.8	3.3
4	2	27	0.1	0.1

Large doses given as a single injection tended to give mainly small bowel tumours whilst divided doses increased the proportion of large bowel tumours. A regimen of 8 weekly injections of AOM at 8 mg/Kg was as effective as 26 injections at the same dosage. Although DMH is metabolised to AOM and then to MAM [3], in practice MAM is less effective and must be administered at 35 mg/Kg per week. DMAB gives intestinal neoplasms when injected subcutaneously, but the tumours are mainly benign, occur in a relatively small proportion of animals and dosages which give intestinal tumours in 33% of animals give a high proportion of tumours at other sites. The direct acting carcinogens MNU and MNNG can be used in a wide range of rodents, but only give tumours in that part of the bowel exposed to the carcinogen (usually the rectum). Intestinal carcinogens have been reviewed extensively by Shamsuddin [4].

Although there are models for the production of intestinal tumours in rats, mice, guinea pigs and hamsters, most work has been done in rats. Guinea pigs are resistant to DMH and AOM, but intestinal tumours can be induced with MNNG and MNU. Strains of rats differ greatly in their sensitivity to DMH and AOM; Sprague-Dawley rats are sensitive and are therefore most commonly used whilst Wistar rats are much more resistant.

Relevance of the Animal Models

The intestinal tumours produced by AOM or DMH in rats show striking similarities to those arising in humans in histopathology, cell biology and kinetics and in tumour markers. Although the experimental tumours tend to be much more highly antigenic than are human tumours, they tend to produce the same antigens. Similarly they are good models for the initial evaluation of chemotherapeutic agents.

However, there are important problems with respect to the use of the model in determining the role of environmental factors in the aetiology of the tumours. Thus the effect of a dietary manipulation can depend on the nature of the carcinogen, the strain of animal used, the nature of the baseline diet, the age of the animals, the temporal relation between the dietary manipulation and the administration of initiator and the method of termination of the study (e.g. at death of the animal compared with at a predetermined time). All of this means that for any given dietary hypothesis there is at least one animal model which confirms it and at least one which resoundingly refutes it. In setting up the model there are usually inbuilt preconceptions. For example the DMH and AOM-rat models were chosen as "good models" because they showed an effect of diet on the rate of tumour formation [5]. In consequence, it is illogical to use such models to try to confirm relationships between dietary components and the risk of carcinogenesis.

Many improvements in the models could be achieved by standardising on a small range of protocols shown to be of value in aetiological studies; the standardisation should be in terms of (a) strain and sex of the rodent used; (b) age of rodents at the start of the experiment; (c) the type and dose of carcinogen to be given; (d) the regime for the administration of the carcinogen (e.g. single dose, 12 equal weekly doses etc.); (e) the dietary regime during carcinogen administration and that given afterwards; (f) type of feeding (ad lib vs. "meals") etc. In general, large amounts of carcinogen are given in order to achieve quick results but as a consequence of this the adenoma-carcinoma sequence tends to be greatly compressed and the distribution of tumours tends to concentrate on the small intestine and is greatly different from that in humans. The model would be much better if the amount of carcinogen given was decreased to a minimum (so that only 10% of animals developed tumours) even though this would mean that studies would need to be life-long rather than of limited duration and the size of the groups of animals would need to be greater. This would result in a better distribution of tumours along the gastro-intestinal tract and much less liver damage (in many studies using DMH or AOM the animals die of hepatotoxicity from the carcinogen and not as a result of any sequelae of carcinogenesis). In the human there is general agreement that carcinomas arise via the adenoma-carcinoma sequence; the animal model needs to feature the same sequence if it is to be of use in aetiological studies. Finally, it is extremely important to have expert and experienced veterinary support as well as the histopathological, biochemical and toxicological back-up in order to ensure that the results of studies are properly interpreted.

Despite the shortcomings listed, a great deal of work has been carried out on the relationship between dietary fat, dietary fibre and colorectal carcinogenesis. A recent review is that by Wilpart [36].

Dietary Fat and Colorectal Cancer

Reddy et al. [6] showed in 1974 that when rats treated with DMH were fed diets containing 0.5%, 4% or 20% corn oil, 90% of the rats on the high fat diet developed colon tumours compared with 60% of the rats on the low fat diet. Similarly, in 1975 Nigro et al. [7] showed that in rats treated with AOM and fed diets containing either 35% or 5% beef fat, those fed the high fat diet developed twice as many tumours as those fed the low fat diet. Reddy [8] showed that whether rats were treated with AOM, DMH, MAM, DMAB or MNU, the rate of tumour formation was always higher in rats fed 20% fat than in those fed 5% fat, whether the fat was beef fat, corn oil or lard. However, not only the amount but the type of fat is important. Thus Reddy et al. [9] reported that, whilst in the DMH-rat model unsaturated fats were more potent tumour promoters than saturated fats at 5% of calories, the distinction disappeared when 20% of fat was used and both types of fat were equally active.

Table 2. The effect of the type and the amount of fat on the colon tumours induced in AOM-treated rats

		Percentage of animals with tumours		
Dietary fat	Dosage	Adenoma	Carcinoma	Total
Corn oil (PUF*)	5%	10	7	17
	23.5%	14	32	46
Safflower oil (PUF)	5%	7	6	13
	23.5%	14	22	36
Olive oil (MUF**/SF°)	5%	7	3	10
	23.5%	10	3	13
Coconut oil (SF)	23.5%	10	3	13

* PUF= Polyunsaturated fat
** MUF= Monounsaturated fat
° SF= Saturated fat

Table 2 summarizes some of the more recent results of Reddy [8] in which it is clear that the effect of corn oil or safflower oil is very much greater than that of olive oil or coconut oil. They further showed that medium-chain triglycerides had little tumour-promoting effect. Many of the early studies were criticised because of failure to control the total number of calories given and because of the form in which the food was given. Even in 1984 a study was set up in which all of the diets were administered in agar [10]; agar and the carrageenan present in it is known to be a promoter of colon carcinogenesis in the animal model and so the failure to show a supplementary promoting effect of added fat was very difficult to interpret. Table 3 lists some typical more recent studies of the role of fat as a promoter of experimental colon carcinogenesis. The general consensus of the studies to date is that (a) fat promotes colon carcinogenesis in most of the animal models; (b) unsaturated fats are usually (but not always) found to be better than saturated fats as promoters of colon carcinogenesis; (c) trans isomers have been shown to be better promoters than cis isomers in a number of studies, but this still remains to be resolved.

Many studies have gone further to test the bile acid hypothesis of colon carcinogenesis. Nigro [1,2] has reviewed the data to 1985 and concluded that the animal model gives good support for the hypothesis since (a) the bile acids lithocholic and deoxycholic acid delivered per rectum are good promoters of colon carcinogenesis in rats treated with AOM, DMH, MNNG and MNU; (b) surgical or experimental procedures which divert increased amounts of bile to the colon increase the number of tumours and *vice versa*; and (c) dietary changes which increase the faecal bile acid concentration also increase the numbers of tumours formed in rats treated with AOM or DMH or MNNG. In a number of recent studies this has been confirmed [e.g. 15,17] and the toxic effect of bile acids on the colonic mucosa [18,19,20] reversed by treatment of the animals with calcium salts delivered orally or per rectum [21,22,23].

Table 3. Recent studies of fat and experimental colon carcinogenesis

Reference	Model	Observation
11	AOM/rats	Unsaturated fats give more tumours and greater malignant differentiation than saturated fats
12	DMH/rats	Used a strict pair-feeding protocol to show that fat promotes colon carcinogenesis. Cellulose either decreased (unsaturated fat) or abolished (saturated fat) this promotion
13	DMH/rats	Trans fatty acids are good promoters but cis isomers are less good
14	AOM/rats	Unsaturated fats increase number of tumours to a greater extent than saturated fats
15	DMH/rats	Fat promoted colon carcinogenesis; effect reversed by fibre
16	DMH/rats	Cis and trans forms equally good promoters
17	AOM/rats	Corn oil and trans fats good promoters; give a dose-response relationship for both

Dietary Fibre and Colorectal Cancer

The situation to 1985 has been reviewed by Kritchevsky [24] and was shown to be extremely confused. In contrast to the observations with fat, the question of whether fibre is protective and, if so, which forms of fibre are most potent receives an answer which is dependent on the exact model used. Thus has been shown to be protective, promoting or inactive in animal models differing only in the carcinogen used. Nigro and Bull [2] concluded that bran and cellulose protect against experimental colon carcinogenesis provided that the diets are formulated correctly and that the amount of fat in the diet is low; in their experience, when bran and cellulose had a protective effect the stool bulk was increased

Table 4. The effect of type of fibre, initiating carcinogen and sex of the rats on experimental colon carcinogenesis

Type of fibre	Rat Model			Effect	Reference
	Carcinogen	Route	Sex of rats		
Cellulose (20% or 40%)	AOM	Sc	M	None	25
Cellulose	DMH	Sc	M	Protect	12
Cellulose 15%	DMH	Oral	M	None	24
Hemicellulose	DMH	Sc	M	None	26
Hemicellulose	DMH	Oral	M	Protect	24
Bran (20%)	DMH	Oral	M	Protect	24
Bran (20%)	DMH	Sc	M	None	24
Bran	DMH	Sc		Promote	27
Bran (20%)	DMH	Oral	F	None	24
Carrot (20%)	DMH	Sc	M	Promote	24
Pectin (15%)	DNU	IR	F	None	25
Pectin (15%)	AOM	Sc	F	Protect	25
Pectin	DMH	Sc	M	Promote	28

2 to 3 fold and the faecal bile acid concentration decreased accordingly. Table 4 illustrates the effect of carcinogen and type of fibre on tumour formation in rats [24]. Hemicellulose was shown to be protective by Watanabe et al. [25] whilst Freeman et al. [26] showed that it merely delayed the time of appearance of the tumours and did not affect the eventual number. Cellulose has been shown to have no effect on experimental carcinogenesis by a number of groups whilst Nigro et al. [1,2] have shown that it is protective if the amount of dietary fat is low and Trudel et al. [12] showed that cellulose protects against the promoting effects of saturated fats but less so against that of unsaturated fat. In male Fisher rats bran is protective against tumours induced by AOM but not against those from MNU [25]. Similarly, in Fisher rats bran is protective against tumours induced by DMH in male but not in female animals [24]. Clearly, therefore, if you believe that bran is good for you there are experimental studies to support you; if you are sceptical there are plenty of studies to support that view as well.

There have been many studies relating the effect of fibre to the faecal bile acids; in general these studies support the hypothesis that where fibre decreases the faecal bile acid concentration it also decreases the number of tumours [1,2,14,15,22-24].

Breast Cancer

The evidence from experimental studies of breast cancer is less confused than that for colorectal cancer, probably because the number of groups studying the subject is fewer and so the multiplicity and variety of protocols is very much smaller.

The Animal Models

In early studies Tannenbaum [29,30] used strains of rats in which there was a high rate of spontaneous carcinogenesis. Later investigations were carried out using rats in which mammary tumours had been induced with dimethylbenzanthracene (DMBA). Semipurified diets are used to which can be added the relevant amounts and types of test components. The subject has been reviewed by Carroll [31,32] and by Cohen [37] together with the data on the effects of diet on tumorigenesis.

Dietary Fat and Mammary Cancer

In early studies [29,30] the rate of development of spontaneous mammary cancers was shown to be increased by high calories and a high fat diet; this was confirmed using the DMBA model [33] and using corn oil as the fat source, but coconut oil gave no increase in tumour yield. The effect of fat on tumour yield was independent of the effect of increased calorie intake. In general, later studies tended to show that polyunsaturated fatty acids increased the yield of mammary tumours whilst saturated fat alone had little effect on tumour yield [31]. When even a small amount of polyunsaturated fat was added to saturated fat, good tumour promotion was oberved, and so early observations of promotion by saturated fat were presumably due to the presence of unsaturated impurities in the fat [31]. Enhancement of tumour yield can be achieved even if there is a time gap between initiation and the commencement of the high fat diet [34]. A change from a high fat to a low fat diet during the study period decreases the tumour yield [35], and so the effect of fat appears to be promotional rather than initiating.

Other work of Carroll and co-workers [see reviews 31,32] has confirmed that fat has its primary action in the post-initiation stage of mammary carcinogenesis. It has also been shown to have a role in tumour initiation, however [38], and alters the development of the mammary gland [39] as well as the hepatic carcinogen-metabolising systems [40]. Various mechanisms have been proposed for the promotional effect of fat in the rat model and these have been discussed in detail by Cohen [37].

There has been considerable interest in the effects of various types and sources of fats in addition to the simple comparison of saturated, unsaturated and polyunsaturated fats. Olive oil (which consists of over 75% oleic acid) was shown to lack tumour promoting activity in the rat model in which NMU was used as the initiator [41] but was a good promoter in the DMBA induced tumour model [31]. Medium chain triglycerides had no tumour promoting effect in the NMU model [42], whilst the polyunsaturated fish oils such as the eicosapentenoic acid fats have been shown to be tumour promoters by one group [43] and to have no effect by another group [44]. These studies are of great importance because of the relation between the results with the animal model and human epidemiology. Populations consuming olive oil have a low incidence of breast cancer, as do populations consuming large amounts of fish. In the attempts to find a more healthy diet the use of fish oil, medium chain triglyceride or of olive oil instead of the fats commonly used in countries with a high incidence of breast cancer might form the basis of recommendations acceptable to the public. It is important, therefore, that the inconsistencies in the findings from the animal models are resolved.

A major problem with the interpretation of the results from the experimental studies is that they are often superficially difficult to reconcile with human epidemiological observations. This was particularly so with respect to the relative importance of saturated and polyunsaturated fat. However, the human diet contains a proportion of polyunsaturated fat which is now known to be sufficient to explain the observed correlation between total fat intake and mammary cancer risk in humans. The animal model of breast cancer appears to be very much more useful than the currently available models of colorectal cancer for the study of aetiological agents.

Dietary Total Calories and Colorectal and Breast Cancer

The effect of total calorie intake in the animal models of breast and colorectal cancer can be discussed together and outside the context of the other dietary factors already reviewed. This is because, whereas in the studies of fat and fibre in colorectal and breast carcinogenesis there are considerable discrepancies in the literature, these are absent from the studies on the effect of calorie intake. In the early studies of Tannenbaum and Silverstone [29,30] it was demonstrated that total calorie intake was associated with cancer risk and this has been confirmed in breast carcinogenesis and in colorectal carcinogenesis. In studies of effects of calorie restriction in has been shown that "under-feeding" of rodents results in a decreased rate of tumour formation at many sites including the breast and large bowel [45]. This effect of under-feeding can be contrasted with the effect of obesity, which is clearly associated with an increased risk of cancer at both sites [47]; this effect is independent of the effect of dietary fat on tumour formation.

REFERENCES

1 Nigro ND: Animal model for colorectal cancer. In: Ingall JR, Mastromarino AJ (eds) Carcinoma of the Large Bowel and its Precursors. Alan Liss 1985: 161-173

2 Nigro ND, Bull AW: Dietary studies of cancer of the large bowel in the animal model. In: Vahouny GV, Kritchevsky D (eds) Dietary Fiber: Basic and Clinical Aspects. New York: Plenum 1986: 467-480

3 Fiala ES: Investigations into the metabolism and mode of action of the colon carcinogens 1,2-dimethylhydroazine and azomethane. Cancer 1977 (4):2436-2445

4 Shamsuddin AKM: In vivo induction of colon cancer. Dose and animal species. In: Autrup H, Willimas GM (eds) Experimental Colon Carcinogenesis. Boca Raton: CRC 1983: 51-62

5 Reddy BS, Narisawa T, Maronpot R, Weisburger JH, Wynder EL: Animal models for the study of dietary factors and cancer of the large bowel. Cancer Res 1975 (35):3421-3426

6 Reddy BS, Weisburger JH, Wynder EL: Effects of dietary fat level and dimethylhydrazine on fecal acid and neutral sterol excretion and colon carcinogenesis in rats. J Natl Cancer Inst 1974 (52):507-511

7 Nigro ND, Singh DV, Campbell RL, Pak MS: Effects of dietary beef fat on intestinal tumour formation by azoxymethane in rats. J Natl Cancer Inst 1975 (54):439-442

8 Reddy BS: Colon Cancer: Future directions. In: Vahouny GV, Kritchevsky D (eds) Dietary Fiber: Basic and Clinical Aspects. New York : Plenum 1986: 543-552

9 Reddy BS, Narisawa T, Vukusich D, Weisburger JH, Wynder EL: Effect of quality and quantity of dietary fat and dimethylhydrazine in colon carcinogenesis in rats. Proc Soc Exp Biol Med 1976 (151):237-239

10 Nauss KM, Locniskoor M, Newberne PM: Effects of alterations in the quality and quantity of dietary fat on 1,2-dimethylhydrazine-induced colon tumorigenesis in rats. Cancer Res 1983 (43):4083-4090

11 Sakaguchi M, Hiramatsu Y, Takada H, Yamamura M, Hioki K, Saito K, Yamamoto M: Effect of dietary unsaturated and saturated fats on azoxymethane-induced colon carcinogenesis in rats. Cancer Res 1984 (44):1472-1477

12 Trudel JL, Senterman MK, Brown RA: The fat fiber antagonism in experimental colon carcinogenesis. Surgery 1983 (94):691-696

13 Hogan AM, Shamsuddin AKM: Large intestinal carcinogenesis. I. Promotional effect of dietary fatty acid isomers in the rat model. J Natl Cancer Inst 1984 (73):1293-1296

14 Sakaguchi M, Minoura T, Hiramatsu Y, Takada H, Yamamura M, Hoika K, Yamamoto M: Effect of dietary saturated and unsaturated fatty acids on fecal bile acids and colon carcinogenesis induced by azoxymethane in rats. Cancer Res 1986 (46):61-65

15 Galloway DJ, Owen RW, Jarrett F: Experimental colon cancer: The relationship of diet and faecal bile acids concentration to tumour induction. Br J Surgery 1986 (73):233-237

16 Watanabe M, Koga T, Sugano M: Influence of dietary cis- and trans-fat on 1,2-dimethylhydrazine-induced colon tumors and fecal steroid excretion in Fisher 344 rats. Am J Clin Nutr 1985 (42):475-484

17 Reddy BS, Tanaka T, Simi B: Effect of different levels of dietary trans fat or corn oil on azoxymethane-induced colon carcinogenesis in F344 rats. J Natl Cancer Inst 1985 (75):791-798

18 Craven PA, Pfanstiel J, Saito R, DeRubertis PR: Relationship between loss of rat colonic surface epithelium induced by deoxycholate and initiation of the subsequent proliferative response. Cancer Res 1986 (46):5754-5759

19 Reiss B, Weiss CJ, Tanaka T, Reddy B, Williams GM: Effects of bile acids on carcinogen-exposed rat colon in organ culture and as subsequent long-term transplants. J Natl Cancer Inst 1987 (78):107-114

20 Suzuki K, Bruce WR: Increase by deoxycholic acid of the colonic nuclear damage induced by known carcinogens in C57BL/6 mice. J Natl Cancer Inst 1986 (76):1129-1132

21 Buset M, Lipkin M, Winawer S, Swaroop S, Friedman E: Inhibition of human colonic epithelial cell proliferation in vivo by calcium. Cancer Res 1986 (46):5426-5430

22 Bird RP, Schneider R, Stamp D, Bruce WR: Effect of dietary calcium and cholic acid on the proliferative indices of murine colonic epithelium. Carcinogenesis 1986 (7):1656-1661

23 Rafter J, Eng V, Furrer R, Medline A, Bruce WR: Effects of calcium and pH on the mucosal damage produced by deoxycholic acid in the rat colon. Gut 1986 (27):1320-1329

24 Kritchevsky D: Fiber and cancer. In: Vahouny G, Kritchevsky D (eds) Dietary Fiber: Basic and Clinical Aspects. New York: Plenum 1986: 427-432

25 Watanabe K, Reddy BS, Weisburger JH, Kritchevsky D: Effect of dietary alfalfa, pectin and wheat bran on azoxymethane- or methylnitrosourea-induced colon carcinogenesis in F344 rats. J Natl Cancer Inst 1979 (63):141-145

26 Freeman HJ, Spiller GA, Kim YS: Effect of high hemicellulose corn-bran in 1,2-diemthylhydrazine-induced rat intestinal neoplasia. Carcinogenesis 1984 (5):261-264

27 Jacobs LR: Stimulation of rat colonic crypt cell proliferative activity by wheat bran consumption during the stage of 1,2-dimethylhydrazine administration. Cancer Res 1984 (44):2458-2463

28 Bauer HG, Asp N, Oste R, Dahlquist A, Fredlund P: Effect of dietary fiber on the induction of colorectal tumours and ß-glucuronidase activity in the rat. Cancer Res 1979 (39):3752-3756

29 Tannenbaum A: The genesis and growth of tumours. III. Effects of a high fat diet. Cancer Res 1942 (2):468-475

30 Silverstone H, Tannenbaum A: The effect of the proportion of dietary fat on the rate of formation of mammary carcinoma in mice. Cancer Res 1950 (10):448-453

31 Carroll KK: Diet and breast cancer - experimental approaches. In: Joossens J, Hill M, Geboers J (eds)

Diet and Human Carcinogenesis. Amsterdam: Excerpta Medica 1985: 265-273
32 Carroll KK: Diet and mammary carcinogenesis. In: Vahouny G, Kritchevsky D (eds) Dietary Fiber: Basic and Clinical Aspects. New York: Plenum 1986: 433-440
33 Carroll KK, Khor HT: Dietary fat in relation to tumorigenesis. Prog Biochem Pharmacol 1975 (10):308-353
34 Hopkins GL, Carroll KK: J Natl Cancer Inst 1979 (62):1009-1012
35 Kalamegham R, Carroll KK: Reversal of the promotional effect of high-fat diet on mammary tumorigenesis by subsequent lowering of dietary fat. Nutr Cancer 1984 (6):22-31
36 Wilpart M: Dietary fats and fibre and experimental colon carcinogenesis: a critical review of published evidence. In: Faivre J, Hill M (eds) Causation and Prevention of Colorectal Cancer. Amsterdam: Excerpta Medica 1987: 85-98
37 Cohen LA: Dietary fat and mammary cancer. In: Reddy BS, Cohen LA (eds) Diet, Nutrition and Cancer: A Critical Review. Boca Raton: CRC Press 1986: 78-100
38 Dao TL, Chan PC: Effect of duration of high fat intake on enhancement of mammary carcinogenesis in rats. J Natl Cancer Inst 1983 (71):201-205
39 Abraham S, Hillyard LA: Lipids, lipogenesis and the effects of dietary fat on growth of mammary tumour model systems. In: Perkins EG, Visek WJ (eds) Dietary Fats and Health. Chamaign: AOCS 1983: 817-852
40 Hopkins GJ, West CE: Effect of dietary fats on pentobarbitone-induced sleeping times and hepatic microsomal P-450 in rats. Lipids 1976 (11):736-740
41 Cohen LA, Thompson DO: Dietary fat, serum lipids and the development of N-nitrosomethylurea-induced mammary tumours. Fed Proc 1984 (43):614
42 Cohen LA, Thompson DO, Maoura Y, Weisburger JH: The influence of dietary medium chain triglycerides on the development of NMU-induced mammary tumors. Cancer Res 1984 (44):5023-5028
43 Carroll KK, Hopkins GJ, Kennedy TG, Davidson MB: Essential fatty acids in relation to mammary carcinogenesis. Prog Lipid Res 1982 (20):685-690
44 Jurkowski JJ, Cave WT: Dietary effects of a N-3 polyunsaturated lipid (Menhaden oil) on the growth and membrane composition of rat mammary tumours. Proc Am Ass Cancer Res 1984 (25):211
45 Tucker MJ: The effect of long term food restriction on tumours in rodents. Int J Cancer 1979 (23):803-807
46 Kritchevsky D, Weber MM, Buck CL, Klurfeld DM: Calories, fat and cancer. Lipids 1986 (21):272-274
47 Waxler SH, Bricker G, Beal SL: The effect of a fat enriched diet on the incidence of spontaneous mammary tumours in obese mice. Proc Soc Exp Biol Med 1979 (162):365-368

Vitamins, Minerals and Other Dietary Factors

A.B. Miller

Department of Preventive Medicine and Biostatistics, University of Toronto, Toronto, Ontario, M5S 1A8, Canada

Introduction

In this chapter, several dietary factors not specifically considered in the other chapters are reviewed. In the main these are what others describe as micronutrients, in contradistinction to the macronutrients (fat, fibre, carbohydrates, protein). Also included are some beverages (coffee, tea). No attempt has been made to be all-inclusive, only those constituents of diet for which there is some epidemiological evidence are considered. Thus, contaminants of food present in trace amounts, e.g. pesticides, are not considered, as the scanty epidemiologic evidence available relates to exposure in the occupational setting, and not in relation to diet. Similar considerations apply to food colouring agents and food preservatives. Aflatoxin is, however, considered as evidence has been accumulating on its association with primary liver cancer in Africa and Asia.

The Vitamins

Vitamin A and Beta-carotene

Lung cancer

Interest in diet and lung cancer began with a cohort study in Norway which showed that an index of vitamin A intake was negatively associated with lung cancer incidence [1,2]. Others had similar findings [3,4].

With a finding of a negative association of beta-carotene but not preformed vitamin A with lung cancer incidence [5], and some understanding on how beta-carotene might be protective [6], attention shifted to beta-carotene. Several authors have found evidence of protective effects of beta-carotene [7-11]. Further, some of the strongest associations in earlier work were with "vitamin A" indices derived from plant foods. Others had also found evidence of a protective effect of vegetables on lung cancer [10,12,13]. However, it cannot be assumed that all, if any, of the protective effect comes from beta-carotene, as many inhibitors of carcinogenesis come from vegetables (see below). Whether or not vegetable consumption rather than pure beta-carotene consumption is protective will be clarified when results from several ongoing chemoprevention trials are available.

All investigators have been careful to adjust their analyses for smoking. Several have also attempted to evaluate interaction with smoking. In one study the reduced relative risk of lung cancer associated with vitamin A was most evident among men who smoked heavily [2]. Hirayama [13] suggested that green-yellow vegetable consumption might hasten the effect of cessation of cigarette smoking, and might also affect the risk due to passive smoking. Samet et al. [8] found effects only in Anglos rather than Hispanics, and only in former rather than current cigarette smokers. Ziegler et al. [10] found the protective effect of vegetables was limited to current and recent cigarette smokers. Pisani et al. [14] found an increased risk of lung cancer for smokers who did not consume carrots, but no corresponding effect for ex- or non-smokers. Byers et al. [11] found the risk reduction associated with vitamin A from fruits and vegetables was most evident for light or ex-smokers. Bond et al. [15] found the strongest inverse association of a vitamin A index with lung cancer risk among cigarette smokers.

Some investigators have also attempted to evaluate differential risks according to histological type. Several found associations that were strongest for squamous cell cancer [4,10,11,16]. Byers et al. [16] also found associations with small cell cancer, and Ziegler et al. [10] with adenocarcinoma for current and recent smokers.

Cancers other than Lung

A case-control study of gastrointestinal cancer in Norway and Minnesota found an inverse association with intake of foods having vitamin A activity [17]. A case-control study of oesophageal cancer in France found evidence of increase in risk with increase in beta-carotene intake [18]. Another case-control study in Pennsylvania also found a weak inverse association between intake of such foods and risk of death from stomach cancer [19]. Risch et al. [20] found an inverse association of beta-carotene with stomach cancer, but this association did not persist in the final model when dietary fibre was included. Graham et al. [21] found no association between intake of foods with vitamin A activity and gastrointestinal cancers. However, they did find that intake of such foods was inversely associated with cancers of the bladder, mouth, larynx, oesophagus and breast, and was positively associated with cancer of the prostate [22].

A hospital-based case-control study in Italy found that intake of dietary beta-carotene, but not of retinol, was inversely associated with risk of invasive cervical cancer after adjustment for risk factors such as age at first intercourse, number of sexual partners, and educational status [23]. This result has been supported by two case-control studies in the U.S. [24,25]. A 5-year prospective study of 1,271 Massachusetts residents 66 years of age or older found an inverse association between frequency of eating green and yellow vegetables and risk of death from cancer [26]. A case-control study in Israel found a strong inverse association between the frequency of consumption of carotene-containing foods and risk of gastro-intestinal cancers [27]. However, the investigators concluded that the association was probably due to factors other than beta-carotene.

Three case-control studies have found a positive association between intake of foods with vitamin A activity and risk of cancer of the prostate [22,28]; Kolonel et al. [29] found a positive association for men aged 70 or older, but not for younger men. However, in a cohort study no statistically significant associations between concentration of serum beta-carotene and 10-year risk of cancers of the colon, stomach, rectum, and urinary bladder were found [30].

In one study, dietary supplementation with retinol and beta-carotene markedly decreased the proportion of micronucleated buccal mucosal cells in Filipino betel chewers [31].

B Vitamins

Deficiencies of riboflavin have been associated in several studies with oesophageal cancer [32-34]. Low levels of riboflavin, vitamin A and carotenoids were found in a population with a high incidence of oral and oesophageal cancer [35]. Endoscopic studies of populations at high risk of oesophageal cancer in China have also found evidence of riboflavin deficiency [36]. However, a one-year intervention trial in a high risk population in China found no evidence of a reduction in prevalence of dysplasia or oesophagitis following weekly supplements of retinol, riboflavin and zinc [37]. Micronuclei were reduced, however [38]. Niacin deficiency has also been associated with oesophageal cancer [33,34,39].

Although pernicious anaemia has been associated with gastric carcinoma, the association is probably due to the gastritis and not to the vitamin B12 deficiency *per se*.

Vitamin C

Meinsma [40] noted that the consumption of citrus fruits by persons with gastric cancer was lower than that by controls. Similar inverse associations between fresh fruit consumption or vitamin C intake and gastric cancer have been reported [43-45]. Risch et al. [20], in a case-control study of stomach cancer conducted in Canada, found that citrus fruit intake appeared to be somewhat protective, while vitamin C intake in a univariate analysis was significantly protective. However, in a logistic regression model simultaneously including multiple factors, vitamin C intake did not make a significant contribution to risk over and above a protective effect for dietary fibre.

Mettlin et al. [46] found inverse associations of indices of vitamin A and vitamin C consumption. The relationship was stronger for vitamin C than for vitamin A, and only the association with vitamin C was statistically significant after controlling for smoking and alcohol use. In studies of oesophageal cancer conducted in the Caspian littoral of Iran, inverse associations were found between oesophageal cancer and consumption of fresh fruits and estimated intake of vitamin C based on correlational and case control data [43-45,47]. In a study of diet and oesophageal cancer conducted in the Calvados region of France, Tuyns et al. [19] found further evidence for a protective effect of vitamin C consumption. Similar protective effects, however, were found for vitamin E and some other micronutrients. It is not clear from this study whether this reflects general nutritional deficiency, particularly in individuals with high alcohol consumption, or possibly a more specific effect of vitamin C.

Jain et al. [48] found no association between vitamin C consumption and colon cancer in a case-control study in Canada. In a case-control study on colorectal cancer in Marseilles a significant protective effect of vitamin C was found after adjustment for age, calories and weight [49]. However, in a multivariate analysis in a model including other macro- or micronutrients, vitamin C was no longer significantly protective. Vitamin C was also evaluated in two case-control studies of colorectal cancer in Australia. In one [50], vitamin C consumption appeared to be associated with a reduced relative risk for rectal cancer in males and females. No protective effect was found for colon cancer. In the other [51], vitamin C was protective for colorectal cancer at the highest consumption level. In another case-control study conducted in Belgium [52], there appeared to be no indication of a protective effect of vitamin C.

The effect of vitamin C has also been assessed in a number of studies of other cancer sites. In a case-control study of laryngeal cancer, Graham et al. [53] found an inverse relationship between risk and indices of both vitamin C and A consumption after controlling for cigarette smoking and alcohol consumption. There was a similar relationship for vegetable consumption in general. An association between vitamin C consumption and uterine cervical dysplasia was reported in a case-control study in New York [54]. The findings persisted after the investigators controlled for sexual activity. Stahelin et al. [55] evaluated plasma vitamin C in a cohort study of over 4,000 men primarily studied for the risk of cardiovascular disease. Plasma vitamin C was found to be consistently lower in cancer cases than in controls. The largest differences were for lung cancer and stomach cancer. Böing et al. [56] analyzed regional data from a national survey on income and food consumption in the Federal Republic of Germany and correlated mortality rates with food consumption data for 15 nutrients. Significant positive correlations were found between vitamin C and cancers of the breast, prostate, liver and colon; for stomach cancer the correlations were negative but not significant. In a case-control study of lung cancer in Hawaii, Hinds et al. [7] found no association between dietary vitamin C intake and lung cancer risk.

In summary, for a number of different cancer sites, indices of vitamin C intake have been found to be associated with a protective effect. The evidence seems strongest for stomach cancer and slightly less so for oesophageal cancer, but is inconsistent for cancers of the colon, rectum and lung. In many studies vitamin C and beta-carotene intake are highly correlated, and it is not certain which, of a number of potential protective factors in foods such as fruits and vegetables, is relevant.

Vitamin E

The possibility that vitamin E (alpha-tocopherol) is protective against some cancers has been suggested by some cohort studies

that had collected and stored serum specimens that were subsequently measured.
Wald [57] found an elevated risk of breast cancer in the lowest quintile of vitamin E plasma samples in a nested case-control study set in a cohort of Guernsey women. Menkes and Comstock [58] found lower vitamin E levels among people who subsequently developed lung cancer than among controls. However, in other studies, little or no difference for cancers of various sites and controls was found [30,55,59]. Salonen et al. [60] noted no differences when vitamin E levels were assessed on their own. There was, however, a strong interaction between vitamin E and selenium. The relative risk of fatal cancer for persons in the lower tertile of selenium and of tocopherol was elevated. Nevertheless, in a further cohort study in Finland, a high serum alpha-tocopherol level was associated with a reduced risk of cancer [61]. The association was strongest for the combined group of cancers unrelated to smoking. The association persisted when adjusted for serum cholesterol, serum vitamin A and serum selenium.
Vitamin E is an antioxidant and free radical scavenger in the lipid phase (whereas vitamin C has similar activity in the acqueous phase) and these effects could be responsible for an anticarcinogenic effect. However, at present the evidence for a protective effect is inconsistent.

Vegetable Intake

In the sections above, several studies that considered the possible protective effect of vegetable-derived indices of vitamin intake, have been reviewed. Several others considered intake in terms of fibre-containing foods, and found evidence of a protective effect against colorectal cancer. The latter studies are reviewed by Jensen (this volume). This section will consider those studies relating fruit or vegetable consumption to cancer risk that were not specifically interpreted in relation to fibre, vitamin A, beta-carotene or vitamin C intake.
In a case-control study of colorectal cancer, Graham et al. [62] found evidence of a protective effect of cabbage and of other vegetables of the *brassica* genus. The protective effects seemed to be particularly related to the frequent ingestion of raw vegetables, especially cabbage, brussels sprouts and broccoli. Haenszel et al. [63] also found an inverse association for cabbage consumption in a case-control study of colorectal cancer in Japan.
These associations were interpreted as a possible effect of inhibition of the microsomal mono-oxygenase system and thus inhibit the activation of chemical carcinogens [64]. In a subequent case-control study of colorectal cancer, Miller et al. [65] found only weak evidence of a protective effect of such vegetables after taking account of saturated fat intake, and then only in females, without a dose-response relationship.
In several studies of lung cancer, evidence of a protective effect of consumption of vegetables has been found [10,12,13]. These studies have generally been interpreted as providing further evidence for a protective effect of beta-carotene. However, it is possible that other factors found in the vegetables may be responsible for some of the protective effect. Indeed, in the cohort study of Hirayama [13] a protective effect of green-yellow vegetable consumption was found for several cancers, including cancers of the stomach and colon, as well as for lung cancer.
In summary, there is consistent evidence of protective effects of fruit and vegetable consumption against several cancers. Although much of this effect could be due to components of dietary fibre (for colo-rectal cancer), vitamin C (for stomach cancer), and beta-carotene (for lung cancer), the possibility remains that other protective factors in vegetables may be responsible for at least part of the protective effects.

Calcium

Calcium reduces the loss of the superficial epithelial cells and/or the compensatory proliferation of the more basal crypt cells which occurs in animals exposed to bile and fatty acids or given excess fat in the diet [66-69]. These dietary effects were seen following concentrations of calcium from 0.1 to 1% by weight of the diet. These levels are higher than would normally be experienced in human diets. Two studies have not shown an effect of calcium on the number of colon tumours but these studies did not demonstrate a large promoting effect of fat [70].

Effects of calcium supplementation on the proliferation of colonic cells in patients considered to be at increased risk for colon cancer have been reported [71]. Calcium carbonate supplementation at 1.2 grams a day led to a reduced colonic crypt labelling pattern with tritiated thymidine that approximated that of a low risk population.

Epidemiological studies have also studied the possibility that dietary calcium influences risk of colon cancer. In a cohort study, the dietary intake of calcium and vitamin D of individuals developing colon cancer was significantly lower than that of individuals without the disease over a follow-up period of 19 years [72]. Those developing the disease had a mean intake of 290 milligrams per day while the intake of the controls was 328 milligrams per day. However, in another cohort study involving a follow-up of 8006 Japanese men in Hawaii, no association between estimated dietary calcium intake and colon cancer risk was found [73].

Dietary calcium intake has been estimated in a number of case control studies of colorectal cancer. No association was found in a reanalysis of a case-control study in Canada [74]. However, a suggestion of a protective effect of calcium with increasing intake was found in a case-control study in Marseille [49]. The risk for the highest consumption category relative to the lowest was 0.7, but the association just failed to achieve statistical significance. In a case control study conducted in Belgium, however, using a similar questionnaire, no association between calcium intake and risk of colorectal cancer was found [52]. In a case-control study conducted in Melbourne, Australia [51], there appeared to be no effect of dietary calcium for males and only a suggestion of a protective effect for high intake in females.

To date, colon cancer and calcium have not been specifically evaluated in international correlation studies. However, it should be noted that some of the comparisons between rural Finland and other parts of Scandinavia or New York, which have been interpreted as showing a protective effect of dietary fibre, could be explained by differences in calcium intake. Although in these studies [75-77] it was found that total fat intake was similar in the areas compared, whereas dietary fibre intake was lower in the high risk area, the main contributer to dietary fat intake in the low risk areas was milk and milk products. Hence, it is likely that the calcium intake in those areas was high. In a study of dietary calcium intake and colon cancer mortality, the crude correlation for 38 countries between these variables was 0.51, colon cancer risk being associated with increased calcium consumption, however [78]. When the results were adjusted for the intake of fat there was a negative correlation of 0.05 but this result depended largely on the influence of Finland.

One study evaluated dietary calcium in relation to risk of oesophageal cancer [19]. A suggestion of a protective effect was found but this was not statistically significant and was substantially less than the protective effect found, for example, from vitamin C.

In conclusion, therefore, although there is strong experimental evidence in animals that dietary calcium may be protective for colon cancer, the evidence from epidemiology is at best inconclusive. One possible explanation for this could be that the levels of dietary calcium in human diets are too low to demonstrate a protective effect.

Selenium

Early correlational studies indicated that a relative deficiency of selenium in the diet might increase the risk of human cancer [79-82]. In an analysis of mortality by county in the United States, in which adjustment was also included for such factors as degree of urbanization, ethnicity and mean annual sunlight, inverse associations of selenium in crops with mortality for all cancer and for lung, colon, rectum, bladder, oesophagus, pancreas, female breast, ovary and cervix cancers were found [83]. For liver, stomach, Hodgkin`s disease and leukemia, however, positive associations were found.

Schrauzer et al. [84] estimated per capita selenium intakes for more than 20 countries based on food disappearance data and found an inverse association between consumption levels and mortality from leukemia and certain cancers. Other correlation studies found inverse associations between selenium levels in pooled blood samples and total cancer mortality as well as mortality from various sites [84,85].

Several investigators have compared blood selenium levels in cancer patients with the corresponding levels in controls [86-97]. In general, these studies found lower levels of selenium in patients than in controls for all cancers combined, as well as for cancers of selected sites.

Several studies based on cohorts with stored prediagnostic serum available from cancer cases and matched controls have been performed. Two studies were carried out in Finland, where selenium intakes are low due to low selenium content in soils. Both found significantly lower selenium levels in patients than controls for all cancers combined [60,98]. In one of these studies, the risk was found to be restricted to men, particularly smokers [60].

In a study in the Netherlands, lower selenium intake was found to be significantly associated with increased total mortality from cancer among men only [99]. Willett et al. [100] found an inverse association between serum selenium level and total cancer incidence. The protective effect was apparent only in smokers, in males, and in blacks (who had lower selenium levels than whites). These studies suggested that cancers of the respiratory and gastrointestinal tracts were most influenced by selenium. In contrast, a positive association between selenium level and cancer risk, especially squamous cell carcinomas, has been found [58]. In addition, Goodwin et al. [90] found higher selenium concentrations in the plasma of patients with cancers of the oral cavity and oropharynx than in controls.

Some studies suggest interaction of selenium with other micronutrients. Thus enhancement of selenium-associated risk by low serum retinol and vitamin E has been found [100], as has enhancement by low vitamin E but not retinol [98]. As the selenium content of foods can vary greatly, estimates of selenium consumption from dietary histories may not reflect individual intake while blood levels can show fluctuations also. Toenail selenium estimation may better reflect actual intake [101].

In summary, various studies suggest that a low intake of selenium or reduced concentrations of selenium in blood or tissues, is associated with increased risk of cancer in man, particularly gastrointestinal sites. However, a firm conclusion on the overall role of selenium in human cancer risk is not yet possible.

Salt

Some investigators reported a positive correlation between occurrence of strokes and gastric cancer mortality [102-105]; stroke occurrence was regarded as a surrogate for salt intake. However, others reported no association [106-108]. Further, cross-sectional and time-trend correlation analyses indicate no association between per capita salt consumption and gastric cancer mortality rates in Japan [109,110]. Nevertheless, higher urinary sodium excretion was found in Columbian populations with elevated gastric cancer mortality rates [111]. Consumption of salted, smoked and pickled fish products or salt-cured ham, sausage and salami was associated with increased gastric cancer risk in blacks in Louisiana [112], in Columbia [113], Europe [114,115], Japan [116-120] and in Japanese in Hawaii [121]. Consumption of salt-containing foods may also account for high rates of gastric cancer in Iceland, Chile, Portugal and the Adriatic coast of Yugoslavia [109,122]. However, salt was not found to be associated with gastric cancer risk in a case-control study in Canada [20].

High salt intake in rodents appears to facilitate both gastric cancer initiation [123,124] and promotion [125-127]. One hypothesis for its role in man is that it facilitates the production of a precursor of gastric cancer, atrophic gastritis [128].

Coffee

Bladder Cancer

Several cohort studies have assessed risk of bladder cancer in relation to coffee consumption. In a cohort study of nearly 24,000 Seventh-Day Adventists, a positive association between deaths from bladder cancer and coffee consumption was found [129]. The association was restricted to those who had never smoked. In contrast, two other large cohort studies, in Norway [130] and in Hawaii [131], failed to find an association.
Two early case-control studies in the United States [132,133] reported elevated risks amongst coffee drinkers, though these were restricted to females in the former study, and black females in the latter study, and there was no evidence of any dose-response relationship. A similar finding was reported from a further case-control study amongst women in Boston [134]. Two other case-control studies, one in Canada [135] and the other in the United States [136], found elevated risks for coffee amongst males, with less evidence for an effect amongst females, though in neither study were dose-response relationships observed. In contrast, no overall effect of coffee drinking was reported in a case-control study carried out in the United States, Britain and Japan [137], in Denmark [138], Japan [139], in a second study in Canada [140] or in a case-control study amongst non-smokers [141]. Three case-control studies, however, have found associations between coffee consumption and risk of bladder cancer, in Greece [142], Connecticut [143] and a 10-centre study in the United States [144]. The Connecticut study found a significant association in males, with some evidence of a dose-response relationship. The 10-centre study, based on nearly 3,000 cases and 6,000 controls, reported a statistically significant overall relative risk of 1.4, but there was no evidence of a dose-response relationship.
Thus, the epidemiologic evidence on coffee drinking and risk of bladder cancer is inconsistent. The fact that even in the positive studies the observed relative risk is small, with no dose-response relationship, suggests that the association is not causal.

Colon Cancer

In the cohort study of nearly 24,000 Seventh-Day Adventists, Snowdon and Phillips [129] found a positive association between coffee consumption and fatal colon cancer. Those consuming 2 or more cups of coffee a day had a relative risk of 1.7 (95% confidence intervals 1.1-2.5) compared to those consuming less than 1 cup a day. This association was restricted to the last 11 years of follow-up, being absent in the first 10 years, and there was a dose-reponse relationship in the latter period, which persisted when meat consumption was included in a multivariate analysis. A significant but small excess risk was found for colon but not rectal cancer in the case-control study of Graham et al. [62]. Nevertheless, in neither of these studies were detailed dietary data collected. It is, therefore, possible that the association with coffee reflects confounding with another factor, such as dietary fat, that could not be evaluated.

Pancreatic Cancer

Although a correlation between coffee drinking and death rates of pancreatic cancer for various countries has been found [145], two large cohort studies, one in the U.S. [146] and the other in Norway [147] failed to find evidence for an association.
In contrast, a case-control study of pancreatic cancer in Boston reported a highly significant dose-response relationship of increasing risk with increasing coffee consumption [148]. However, in a second study carried out by the same authors [149], the association was substantially weaker, and in particular a dose-response relation was not found. Other case control studies [150-153] also failed to find consistent evidence of an association between coffee drinking and risk of pancreatic cancer.

Breast cancer

Three case-control studies, one in Israel [154], one in the United States [155] and one in France [156], have examined evidence for a possible relationship between coffee drinking and risk of breast cancer. All three studies found no evidence of an association.

Ovarian cancer

Two case-control studies, one in Italy [157] and one in Greece [158], found evidence for an association between coffee drinking and increased risk of ovarian cancer. In contrast, two studies in the U.S. and Canada [159,160] failed to find any evidence for this association. Thus the evidence is inconsistent.

Tea

Tea has been negatively associated with pancreatic cancer [148,151,161], though a case-control study using data from England and Wales in the 1950s showed a positive association of tea intake and risk of pancreatic cancer in men [162]. In two of the studies [148,162] hospital controls were used, some or all of whom had cancers of other sites. Potential selection factors among these controls may account for the differences in the results.

Lack of an association between tea consumption and bladder cancer risk has been reported consistently in several studies [135,161,163-166].

A weak negative association between tea intake and prostate cancer was reported in a geographical correlation study [166], and another weak negative association between tea consumption and male liver cancer risk was reported in a cohort study [161].

Tea drinking did not influence the risk of ovarian cancer in a case-control study in the U.S. and Canada [160].

Two case-control studies showed no significant association between tea consumption and colorectal cancer [167,168]. Neither did a Canadian case-control study for consumption of combined beverages (tea, coffee, or colas) [65]. An international geographic correlation study showed a slight negative association with rectal cancer, but a positive association with colon cancer [166]. Heilbrun et al. [161], however, found a positive association of tea consumption and rectal cancer risk over a 16-19 year follow-up period. No risks were reported for any other sites.

Thus, there is no convincing evidence relating tea consumption to any type of cancer.

Artificial Sweeteners

Saccharin

Studies in rodents suggest that the bladder is the target organ for animal carcinogenesis of saccharin. However, population studies [169], and studies of diabetics, who use artificial sweeteners extensively [170,171], have not found associations of bladder cancer with artificial sweetener consumption.

A number of case-control studies of individual use of artificial sweeteners have been reported. Kessler [172,173] found no evidence of any increased risk associated with the use of artificial sweeteners. In contrast, a case-control study from Canada found a statistically significant association in males with the use of artificial sweeteners, primarily saccharin [135,174]. The data also showed a significant dose-response relationship. No effect was found in females. Subsequently, a much larger case control study involving 3,010 cases and 5,783 controls was reported [175]. The results showed no overall increased risk associated with use of artificial sweeteners. However small, statistically significant excess risks were found among subjects who reported use of both table-top artificial sweeteners and diet drinks, with heavy use of one of these.

The great majority of the other case-control studies of bladder cancer and artificial sweetener use [140,176-181] were negative. Some found increased risk in subgroups [140,176,179]. These subgroup findings, however, were not consistent with each other or with the largest study [175]. Thus overall, the epidemiological evidence does not suggest that consumption of saccharin materially increases the risk of bladder cancer.

Cyclamate

Cyclamate was usually given in a 10:1 cyclamate:saccharin mixture and therefore it has rarely been possible to separate the effects of the two substances in studies in the U.S. Thus most of the epidemiologic studies referred to under *Saccharin* relate either to saccharin alone, or to the mixture, until such time as cyclamate was banned in the U.S.

In Canada, however, saccharin was banned as a food and soft drink additive in 1978 but cyclamate use continued. Thus in a recent case-control study in Canada it was possible to separate saccharin and cyclamate use [140]. No consistent increase in risk was found for either males or females.

Nitrate, Nitrite and N-Nitroso Compounds

Nitrate and nitrite are used as preservatives in many foods and can be converted to N-nitroso compounds under a variety of conditions [182]. They can also occur naturally in foods, and because many N-nitroso compounds are strongly carcinogenic in many species [183,184], there has been much concern about their role in the aetiology of human cancer. Because nitrite is present in saliva, and in the urine of people with bladder infections, N-nitroso compounds can be formed in the stomach and bladder from ingested amines, which can be naturally present in food, from residues of agricultural chemicals on food and from drugs and medicines [185].

Epidemiologic studies conducted in several countries showed associations between increased incidence of cancer of the stomach and exposure to high levels of nitrate or nitrite in the diet or drinking water [188-189]. Bladder cancer has been correlated with nitrate in the water supply, or with urinary tract infections [135,190]. Nitrosamines have been found in the urine of patients with urinary tract infections [191]. However, no differences were reported in consumption of nitrite-preserved meats, such as ham or pork sausages, between bladder cancer cases and controls [135].

In China, an increased risk of oesophageal cancer was associated with ingestion of mouldy food containing N-nitroso compounds, possibly produced by fungal contaminants [192]. A correlation has been found between lesions of the oesophageal epithelium and the amount of nitrosamines present in Lin-Xian inhabitants in China [193]. Studies in Iran, however, found no differences in nitrosamine levels in foods in regions of high and low risk for oesophageal cancer [45].

Several studies in different parts of the world have shown an association between frequent consumption of cured pickles or smoked foods and stomach cancer [194-196]. In South Louisiana, consumption of smoked foods and homemade or home-cured meats was found to increase the risk of gastric cancer in the high risk blacks, but not in the lower risk whites [197]. In Canada, consumption of nitrite, smoked meats and smoked fish were found to be risk factors [20]. However, the major contributor to risk was estimated consumption of nitrite.

Thus, it seems likely that consumption of nitrite with endogenous production of nitrosamines makes a major contribution to the risk of stomach cancer.

Aflatoxin

Various studies conducted in Africa and Asia have shown strong correlations between estimated levels of ingested aflatoxin and liver cancer incidence [198].

Oettle [199] suggested that the geographic distribution of liver cancer in Africa could be due to differential exposures to aflatoxin in the diet. Associations between consumption of foods contaminated with aflatoxin and liver cancer in different areas of Swaziland and Uganda have been reported [200,201]. Studies from Swaziland [202,203], from the Muranga district of Kenya [204] and from Mozambique, which has perhaps the highest rates of liver cancer in the world [205,206], have confirmed strong associations between liver cancer incidence and estimated levels of aflatoxin.

In Asia, a correlation between estimated aflatoxin intake and liver cancer incidence in two regions of Thailand was reported [208-209]. In Guangxi province in China and in Taiwan, the frequency of food contamination with aflatoxin has been correlated with liver cancer mortality [210,211]. In several areas of China, food contamination with aflatoxin appears to be a high risk factor for primary liver cancer [212].

A case-control study in the Phillipines determined aflatoxin contamination levels in dietary items and related these to individual consumption [213]. Significantly increased risks of hepatocellular cancer were found for those with high intakes of aflatoxin, with suggestion of a dose-response relationship.

Several studies have shown a high correlation between exposure to hepatitis B virus and primary hepatocellular carcinoma [214-218]. Van Rensberg et al. [206] concluded that preexisting viral infection may be necessary for malignant transformation by aflatoxin.

In three studies, an attempt has been made to take serological evidence of chronic hepatitis B infection into account while evaluating elevated aflatoxin ingestion. In China, aflatoxin levels in both diet and urine were found to be related to hepatocellular incidence, but corresponding differences in the prevalence of hepatitis B carriers was not found [219,220]. In Swaziland liver cancer incidence was strongly associated with estimated levels of aflatoxin in food, with aflatoxin exposure being a more important determinant of liver cancer incidence than hepatitis B infection prevalence in a multivariate analysis [203].

In summary, there is now strong evidence that, in many developing countries, aflatoxin is an important cause of primary liver cancer, probably in conjunction with hepatitis B viral carrier states. There is, however, little or no evidence that aflatoxin intake makes a significant contribution to risk of primary liver cancer, or any other cancer, in Europe.

REFERENCES

1 Bjelke E: Dietary vitamin A and human lung cancer. Int J Cancer 1975 (15):561-565
2 Kvale G, Bjelke E, Gart JJ: Dietary habits and lung cancer risk. Int J Cancer 1983 (31):397-405
3 Mettlin C, Graham S, Swanson MJ: Vitamin A and lung cancer. JNCI 1979 (62):1435-1438
4 Gregor A, Lee PM, Roe FJC et al: Comparison of dietary histories in lung cancer cases and controls with special reference to vitamin A. Nutr Cancer I980 (2):93-97
5 Shekelle RB, Lepper M, Lui S et al: Dietary vitamin A and risk of cancer in the Western Electric Study. Lancet 1981(2):1185-1189
6 Peto R, Doll R, Buckley JD, et al: Can dietary beta-carotene materially reduce human cancer rates? Nature 1981 (290):201-208
7 Hinds MW, Kolonel LN, Hankin HJ et al: Dietary vitamin A, carotene, vitamin C and risk of lung cancer in Hawaii. Am J Epidemiol 1984 (119):227-237
8 Samet JM, Skipper BJ, Humble CG et al: Lung cancer risk and vitamin A consumption in New Mexico..Am Rev Resp Dis 1985 (131):198-202
9 Wu AH, Henderson BE, Pike MC, et al: Smoking and other risk factors for lung cancer in women. JNCI 1985 (74):747-751
10 Ziegler RG, Mason TJ, Stemhagan A et al: Carotenoid intake, vegetables, and the risk of lung cancer among white men in New Jersey. Am J Epidemiol 1986 (123):1080-1093
11 Byers TE, Graham S, Haughey BP et al: Diet and lung cancer risk: findings from the Western New York diet study. Am J Epidemiol 1987 (125):351-363
12 MacLennan R, Da Costa J, Day NE et al: Risk factors for lung cancer in Singapore Chinese, a population with high female incidence rates. Int J Cancer 1979 (20):854-860
13 Hirayama T: Nutrition and cancer - a large scale cohort study. In: Knudsen I (ed) Genetic Toxicology of the Diet. New York: Alan R Liss Inc, 1986 pp 299-311
14 Pisani P, Berrino F, Macaluso M et al: Carrots, green vegetables and lung cancer: a case-control study. Int J Epidemiol 1986 (15):463-468
15 Bond GG, Thompson FE, Cook RR: Dietary vitamin A and lung cancer: results of a case-control study among chemical workers. Nutr Cancer 1987 (9):109-121
16 Byers T, Vena J, Mettlin C et al: Dietary vitamin A and lung cancer risk: an analysis by histologic subtypes. Am J Epidemiol 1984 (120):769-776
17 Bjelke E: Dietary factors and the epidemiology of cancer of the stomach and large bowel. In: Kasper H (ed) Aktuelle Probleme der klinischen Diatetik. Erkrankungen des Verdauungstraktes. Supplement zu Aktuelle Ernahrungsmedizin. Stuttgart: Georg Thieme Verlag,1978 pp 10-17
18 Tuyns AJ, Riboli E, Doornbos G et al: Diet and esophageal cancer in Calvados (France). Nutr Cancer 1987 (9):81-92
19 Stehr PA, Gloninger MF, Kuller LH et al: Dietary vitamin A deficiencies and stomach cancer. Am J Epidemiol 1985 (121):65-70
20 Risch HA, Jain M, Choi NW et al: Dietary factors and the incidence of cancer of the stomach. Am J Epidemiol 1985 (122):947-957
21 Graham S et al: Results of case-control studies of diet and cancer in Buffalo, New York. Cancer Res 1983 (43 Suppl):2409s-2413s
22 Graham S, Humphry B, Marshall J et al: Diet in the epidemiology of carcinoma of the prostate gland. JNCI 1983 (70):687-692
23 La Vecchia C, Franceschi S, Decarli A et al: Dietary vitamin A and the risk of invasive cervical cancer. Int J Cancer 1984 (34):319-322
24 Marshall JR, Graham S, Byers T et al: Diet and smoking in the epidemiology of cancer of the cervix. JNCI 1983 (70):847-851
25 Wylie-Rosett JA, Romney SL, Slagle NS et al: Influence of vitamin A on cervical dysplasia and carcinoma in situ. Nutr Cancer 1984 (6):49-57
26 Colditz GA, Branchl LG, Lipnick RJ et al: Increased green and yellow vegetable intake and lowered cancer deaths in an elderly population. Am J Clin Nutr 1985 (41):32-36
27 Modan B, Cuckle H, Lubin F: A note on the role of dietary retinol and carotene in human gastrointestinal cancer. Int J Cancer 1981 (28):421-424
28 Heshmat MY, Kaul L, Kovi J et al: Nutrition and prostate cancer: a case-control study. Prostate 1985 (6):7-17
29 Kolonel LN, Hankin JN, Yoshizawa CN: Vitamin A and prostate cancer in elderly men: enhancement of risk. Cancer Res 1987 (47):2982-2985
30 Nomura AMY, Stemmerman GN, Heilbrun LK et al: Serum vitamin levels and the risk of cancer of specific sites in men of Japanese ancestry in Hawaii. Cancer Res 1985 (45):2369-2372
31 Stitch HF, Rosin MP, Vallejera MO: Reduction with vitamin A and beta-carotene administration of proportion of micronucleated buccal mucosa cells in Asian betel nut and tobacco chewers. Lancet I984 (1):1204-1206
32 Wynder EL, Bross IJ: A study of etiological factors in cancer of the esophagus. Cancer 1961 (14):389-413
33 van Rensburg SF: Epidemiologic and dietary evidence for a specific nutritional predisposition to esophageal cancer. JNCI 1981 (67):243-251
34 Thurnham DI, Rathakette P, Hambridge KM et al: Riboflavin, vitamin A and zinc status in Chinese subjects in a high-risk area for oesophageal cancer in China. Human Nutr Clin Nutr 1982 (36C):337-349
35 Zaridze DG, Blettner M, Trapeznikov NN et al: Survey of a population with a high incidence of oral and oesophageal cancer. Int J Cancer 1985 (36):153-158
36 Thurnham DI, Zheng SF, Munoz N et al: Comparison of riboflavin, vitamin A, and zinc status of Chinese populations at high and low risk for esophageal cancer. Nutr Cancer I985 (7):131-143

37 Munoz N, Wahrendorf J, Bang LJ et al: No effect of riboflavine, retinol, and zinc on prevalence of precancerous lesions of oesophagus. Lancet 1985 (2):111-114
38 Munoz N, Hayashi M, Bang LJ, Wahrendorf J, Crespi M, Bosch FX: Effect of riboflavin, retinol, and zinc on micronuclei of buccal mucosa and of esophagus: a randomized double-blind intervention study in China. JNCI 1987 (79): 687-691
39 Warwick GP, Harrington JS: Some aspects of the epidemiology and etiology of esophageal cancer with particular emphasis on the Transkei, South Africa. Adv Cancer Res 1973: 81
40 Meinsma L: Nutrition and cancer. Voeding 1964 (25):357-365
41 Higginson J: Etiological factors in gastrointestinal cancer in man. JNCI 1966 (37):527-545
42 Haenszel W, Correa P: Developments in the epidemiology of stomach cancer over the past decade. Cancer Res 1975 (35):3452-3459
43 Cook-Mozaffari P: The epidemiology of cancer of the oesophagus. Nutr Cancer 1979 (1):51-60
44 Cook-Mozaffari PJ, Azordegan F, Day NE et al: Oesophageal cancer studies in the Caspian littoral of Iran: results of a case-control study. Br J Cancer 1979 (39):293-309
45 Joint Iran-International Agency for Research on Cancer Study Group: Esophageal cancer studies in the Caspian littoral of Iran; Results of population studies - A prodrome. JNCI 1977 (59):1127-1138
46 Mettlin C, Graham S, Priore , Marshall J, Swanson M: Diet and cancer of the esophagus. Nutr Cancer 1980 (2):143-147
47 Hormozdiari H, Day NE, Aramesh B, Mahboubi E: Dietary factors and esophageal cancer in the Caspian littoral of Iran. Cancer Res 1975 (35):3493-3498
48 Jain M, Cook GM, Davis FG et al: A case-control study of diet and colo-rectal cancer. Int J Cancer 1980 (26):757-768
49 Macquart-Moulin G, Riboli E, Cornee J et al: Case-control study on colorectal cancer and diet in Marseilles. Int J Cancer 1986 (38):183-191
50 Potter JD, McMichael AJ: Diet and cancer of the colon and rectum: a case-control study. JNCI 1986 (76):557-569
51 Kune S, June GA, Watson LF: Case-control study of dietary etiological factors: The Melbourne Colorectal Cancer Study. Nutr Cancer 1987 (9):21-42
52 Tuyns AJ, Haelterman M, Kaaks R: Colorectal cancer and intake of nutrients; oligosaccharides are a risk factor, fats are not. A case-control study in Belgium. Nutr Cancer 1987 (10):181-196
53 Graham S, Mettlin C, Marshall J et al: Dietary factors in the epidemiology of cancer of the larynx. Am J Epidemiol 1981 (113):675-680
54 Wassertheil-Smoller S, Romney SL, Wylie-Rosett J et al: Dietary vitamin C and uterine cervical dysplasia. Am J Epidemiol 1981 (114):714-724
55 Stahelin HB, Rosel F, Buess E et al: Cancer, vitamins and plasma lipids: prospective Basel study. JNCI 1984 (13):1460-1468
56 Boing H, Martinez L, Frentzel-Beyme R, Oltersdorf U: Regional nutritional pattern and cancer mortality in the Federal Rupublic of Germany. Nutr Cancer 1985 (7):121-130
57 Wald NJ, Boreham J, Haywood JL et al: Plasma retinol, beta-carotine and vitamin E levels in relation to future risk of breast cancer. Br J Cancer 1984 (49):321-324
58 Menkes MS, Comstock GW, Vuilleumier JP et al: Serum beta-carotene, vitamins A and E, and the risk of lung cancer. N Eng J Med 1986 (315):1250-1254
59 Willett WC, Polk BF, Underwood BA et al: Relation of serum vitamins A. and E and carotenoids to the risk of cancer. N Eng J Med 1984 (310):430-434
60 Salonen JR, Salonen R, Lappetelainen R et al: Risk of cancer in relation to serum concentrations of selenium and vitamins A and E: matched case-control analysis of prospective data. Br Med J 1985 (290):417-420
61 Knekt P, Aroma A, Maatela J, Aaran RK, Nikkari T, Hakama M, Hakulinen T, Peto R, Saxen E and Teppo L: Serum vitamin E and risk of cancer among Finnish men during a 10 year follow-up. Am J Epidemiol 1988 (127):28-41
62 Graham S, Dayal H, Swanson M et al: Diet in the epidemiology of cancer of the colon and rectum. JNCI 1978 (61):709-714
63 Haenszel W, Locke FB, Segi M: A case-control study of large bowel cancer in Japan. JNCI 1980 (64):17-22
64 Wattenberg LW: Inhibitors of chemical carcinogens. In: Burchenal JH, Oettgen HF (eds) Cancer: Achievements, Challenges and Prospects for the 1980s. Vol 1. New York: Grune and Stratton, 1981 pp 517-539
65 Miller AB, Howe GR, Jain M et al: Food items and food groups as risk factors in a case-control study of diet and colo-rectal cancer. Int J Cancer 1983 (32):155-161
66 Wargovich MJ, Eng VWS, Newmark HL et al: Calcium ameliorates the toxic effect of decoxycholic acid and colonic epithelium. Carcinogenesis 1983 (4):1205-1207
67 Rafer J, Eng VWS, Furrer R et al: The Effect of Calcium and pH on the mucosal damage produced by deoxycholic acid in the rat colon. Gut 1986 (27):1320-1329
68 Bird RP, Schneider R, Stamp D et al: Effect of dietary calcium and cholic acid on the proliferation indices of murine colon epithelium. Carcinogenesis 1986 (7):1957-1661
69 Bird RP: Effect of dietary components on the pathobiology of colonic epitheliuim: possible relationship with colon tumorigenesis. Lipids 1986 (21):289-291
70 Bull A, Bird RP, Bruce JR, Nigro N, Medline A et al: Effect of calcium on azoxymethane induced intestinal tumors in rats. Abstract Am Gastroenterol Assoc. May 10-13, 1987
71 Lipkin M, Newmark H: Effect of added dietary calcium on colonic epithelial cell proliferation in subjects at high risk for familial colon cancer. New Eng J Med 1985 (313):1381-1384

72 Garland C, Shekelle RB, Barrett-Connor E et al: Dietary vitamin D and calcium and risk of colorectal cancer: A 19-year prospective study in men. Lancet 1985 (1):307-309
73 Heilbrun LK, Hankin JM, Nomura AMY et al: Colon cancer and dietary fat, phosphorus and calcium in Hawaiian-Japanese men. Am J Clin Nutr 1986 (43):306-309
74 Howe GR, Eyssen GM, Miller AB: Calcium intake as a protective factor for large bowel cancer: results of a case-control study. In preparation, 1988
75 International Agency for Research on Cancer Intestinal Microecology Group. Dietary fibre, transit-time, fecal bacteria, steroids and colon cancer in two Scandinavian populations. Lancet 1977 (11):207-211
76 Jensen OM, MacLennan R, Wahrendorf J (On behalf of the IARC large bowel cancer group): Diet, bowel function, fecal characteristics, and large bowel cancer in Denmark and Finland. Nutr Cancer 1982 (4):5-19
77 Reddy BS, Hedges AR, Laakso K, Wynder EL: Metabolic epidemiology of large bowel cancer. Fecal bulk and constituents of high-risk North American and low-risk Finnish population. Cancer 1978 (42):2832-2838
78 Eyssen GM, Bright-See E. 1988. Manuscript in preparation
79 Shamberger RJ, Frost DV: Letter to the Editor: Possible protective effect of selenium against human cancer. Can Med Assoc J 1969 (100):682
80 Shamberger RJ, Willis CE: Selenium distribution and human cancer mortality. CRC Crit Rev Clin Lab Sci 1971 (2):211-221
81 Shamberger RJ, Tytko SA, Willis CE: Antioxidants and cancer. Part VI. Selenium and age-adjusted human cancer mortality. Arch Environ Health 1976 (31):231-235
82 Cowgill UM: The distribution of selenium and cancer mortality in the continental United States. Biological Trace Element Res 1983 (5):345-361
83 Clark LC: The epidemiology of selenium and cancer. Fed Proc 1985 (44):2584-2589
84 Schrauzer GN, White DA, Schneider CJ: Cancer mortality correlation studies - III. Statistical associations with dietary selenium intakes. Bioinorg Chem 1977 (7):23-34
85 Schrauzer GN, White DA and Schneider CJ: Cancer mortality correlation studies - IV. Associations with dietary intakes and blood levels of certain trace elements, notably Se-antagonists. Bioinorg Chem 1977 (7):35-56
86 Broghamer WL Jr, McConnell KP, Blotcky AJ: Relationship between serum selenium levels and patients with carcinoma. Cancer 1976 (37):1384-1388
87 Broghamer WL Jr, McConnell KP, Grimald M et al: Serum selenium and reticuloendothelial tumors. Cancer 1978 (41):1462-1466
88 Calautti P, Moschini G, Stievano BM, Tomio L et al: Serum selenium levels in malignant lymphoproliferative diseases. Scand J Haematol 1980 (24):63-66
89 Clark LC, Graham GF, Crounse RG et al: Plasma selenium and skin neoplasms: a case-control study. Nutr Cancer 1984 (6):12-21
90 Goodwin WJ, Lane HW, Bradford K et al: Selenium and glutathione peroxidase levels in patients with epidermoid carcinoma of the oral cavity and oropharynx. Cancer 1983 (51):110-115
91 McConnell KP, Broghamer WL Jr, Blotcky AJ et al: Selenium levels in human blood and tissues in health and in disease. J Nutr 1975 (105):1026-1031
92 McConnell KP, Jager RM, Bland KI et al: The relationship of dietary selenium and breast cancer. J Surg Oncol 1980 (15):67-70
93 Robinson MF, Godfrey PJ, Thomson CD et al: Blood selenium and glutathione peroxidase activity in normal subjects and in surgical patients with and without cancer in New Zealand. Am J Clin Nutr 1979 (32):1477-1485
94 Schrauzer GN, Molenaar T, Mead S et al: Selenium in the blood of Japanese and American women with and without breast cancer and fibrocystic disease. Jpn J Cancer Res (GANN) 1985 (76):374-377
95 Shamberger RJ, Rukovena E, Longfield AK et al: Antioxidants and cancer. I. Selenium in the blood of normal and cancer patients. JNCI 1973 (50):863-870
96 Sundstrom H, Yrjanheikki E, Kauppila A: Low serum selenium concentration in patients with cervical or endometrial cancer. Int J Gynaecol Obstet 1984 (22):35-40
97 Thimaya S, Ganapath SN: Selenium in human hair in relation to age, diet, pathological condition and serum levels. Sci Total Environ 1982 (24):41-49
98 Salonen JR, Alfthan G, Huttunen JK et al: Association between serum selenium and the risk of cancer. Am J Epidemiol 1984 (120):342-349
99 Kok FJ, de Bruijn AM, Hofman A et al: Is serum selenium a risk factor for cancer in men only? Am J Epidemiol 1987 (125):12-16
100 Willett WC, Morris JS, Pressel S et al: Prediagnostic serum selenium and the risk of cancer. Lancet 1983 (2):130-134
101 Willett W: Nutritional epidemiology: issues and challenges. Int J Epidemiol 1987 (16; Suppl):312-317
102 Joossens JV: Stroke, stomach cancer and salt: a possible clue to the prevention of hypertension. In: Kesteloot H, Joossens JV (eds) Epidemiology of Arterial Blood Pressure. The Hague: Martinus Nijhoff 1980 pp 489-508
103 Joossens JB, Geboers J: Nutrition and gastric cancer. Proc Nutr Soc 1981 (40):37-46
104 Joossens JB, Geboers J: Diet and environment in the etiology of gastric cancer. In: Levin B and Riddell RH (eds) Frontiers of Gastrointestinal Cancer. New York: Elsevier 1984 pp 167-183
105 Tuomilehto J, Geboers J, Joossens JV et al: Trends in stomach cancer and stroke in Finland: comparison to Northwest Europe and USA. Stroke 1984 (15):823-828
106 Harrington JS: Advances in cancer epidemiology in South Africa. S Afr Cancer Bull 1981 (25):9-18
107 Walker AR: Changing disease patterns in South Africa. S Afr Med J 1982 (61):126-129

108 Whelton PK, Goldblatt P: An investigation of the relationship between stomach cancer and cerebrovascular disease: evidence for and against the salt hypothesis. Am J Epidemiol 1982 (115):418-427
109 Howson CP, Hiyama T, Wynder EL: The decline in gastric cancer: epidemiology of an unplanned triumph. Epidemiol Rev 1986 (8):1-27
110 Kono S, Ikeda M, Ogata M: Salt and geographical mortality of gastric cancer and stroke in Japan. J Epid Comm Hlth 1983 (37):43-46
111 Correa P, Montes G, Cuello C et al: Urinary sodium-to-creatinine ratio as an indicator of gastric cancer risk. NCI Monogr 1985 (69):121-123
112 Correa P, Haenszel W, Cuello C et al: A model for gastric cancer epidemiology. Lancet 1975 (2):58-60
113 Correa P, Cuello C, Fajardo LF et al: Diet and gastric cancer: nutrition survey of a high-risk area. JNCI 1983 (70):673-678
114 Bjelke E: Epidemiologic studies of cancer of the stomach, colon, and rectum. Scand J Gastroenterol 1974 (9 Suppl 31):1-235
115 Sato T, Fukuyama T, Suzuki T et al: Studies of the causation of gastric cancer: intake of highly brined foods in several places with high mortality rate in Europe. Jpn Bull Inst Publ Health 1961 (10):9-17
116 Hara J, Sakata K, Nagai M et al: Statistical analyses on the pattern of food consumption and digestive-tract cancers in Japan. Nutr Cancer 1985 (6):220-228
117 Hirayama T: Diet and Cancer. Nutr Cancer 1979 (1):67-81
118 Ishiwata H, Boriboon P, Nakamura Y et al: Studies in vivo formation of nitroso compounds. II. Changes of nitrite and nitrate concentrations in human saliva after ingestion of vegetables on sodium nitrate. J Food Hyg Soc Jpn 1975 (16):19-24
119 Sato T, Fukuyama T, Suzuki T et al: Studies of the causation of gastric cancer. II. The relation between gastric cancer mortality rate and salted food intake in several places in Japan. Jpn Bull Inst Publ Health 1959 (8):187-198
120 Haenszel W, Kurihara M, Segi M et al: Stomach cancer among Japanese in Hawaii. JNCI 1972 (49):969-988
121 Kolonel LN, Hinds MW, Hankin JH: Cancer patterns among migrant and native-born Japanese in Hawaii in relation to smoking, drinking, and dietary habits. In: Gelboin HB, MacMahon B, Matsushmi T et al (eds) Genetic and Environmental Factors in Experimental and Human Cancer. Proceedings of the 10th International Symposium of the Princess Takamatsu Cancer Research Fund (1979). Tokyo: Japan Scientific Societies Press 1980 pp 327-340
122 Alderson M: International mortality statistics. New York: Facts on File Inc 1981
123 Kodama N, Saito H, Yamaizumi Z: Formation of alkylureas in the environment. In: Bartsch H, O'Neill IK, Castegnaro M et al: N-nitroso compounds: occurrence and biological effects. IARC Sci Publ 1982 (41):131-136
124 Takahashi M: Enhancing effect of a high salt diet on gastrointestinal carcinogenesis. Gan No Rinsho 1986 (32):667-673
125 Hanawa K, Yamada S, Suzuki H et al: Effects of sodium chloride on gastric cancer induction by N-methyl-N'-nitro-nitrosoguandine (MNNG) in rats. In: Proceedings of the 39th Annual Meeting of the Japanese Cancer Association. Tokyo: Japanese Cancer Association 1980 p 49
126 Ohgaki H, Kato T, Morion K et al: Study of the promoting effect of sodium chloride on gastric carcinogenesis by N-methyl-N'-nitro-N-nitroso-guanidine in inbred Wistar rats. Gann 1984 (75):1053-1057
127 Takahashi M, Kokubo T, Furukawa F et al: Effect of high salt diet on rat gastric carcinogenesis induced by N-methyl-N'-nitro-N-nitroso-guanidine. Gann 1983 (74):28-34
128 Correa P: Precursors of gastric and esophageal cancer. Cancer 1982 (50):2554-2565
129 Snowdon DA, Phillips RJ: Coffee consumption and risk of fatal concers. Am J Publ Health 1984 (74):820-826
130 Jacobson BD, Bjelke E, Kvale G et al: Coffee drinking mortality, and cancer incidence: results from a Norwegian prospective study. JNCI 1986 (76):823-831
131 Nomura A, Heilbrun LK, Stemmermann GN: Prospective study of coffee consumption and the risk of bladder cancer. JNCI 1986 (76) 587-590
132 Cole P: Coffee drinking and cancer of the lower urinary tract. Lancet 1971 (1):1335-1337
133 Fraumeni JF, Scotto J, Dunham LJ: Coffee drinking and bladder cancer. Lancet 1971 (2):1204
134 Simon D, Yen S, Cole P: Coffee drinking and cancer of the lower urinary tract. JNCI 1975 (54):587-591
135 Howe GR, Burch JD, Miller AB et al: Tobacco use, occupation, coffee, various nutrients, and bladder cancer. JNCI 1980 (64):701-713
136 Mettlin C, Graham S: Dietary risk factors in human bladder cancer. Am J Epidemiol 1979 (110):255-263
137 Morrison AS, Buring JE, Verhoek WG et al: Coffee drinking and cancer of the lower urinary tract. JNCI 1982 (68):91-94
138 Jensen OM, Wahrendorf J, Knudsen JB, Sorenson BL: The Copenhagen case-control study of bladder cancer. II. The effect of coffee and other beverages. Int J Cancer 1986 (37):651-657
139 Ohno Y, Aoki K, Obata K et al: Case-control study of urinary bladder cancer in metropolitan Nagoya. NCI Monogr 1985 (69):229-234
140 Risch HA, Burch JD, Miller AB et al: Dietary factors and the incidence of cancer of the urinary bladder. Am J Epidemiol 1988 (127):1179-1191
141 Kabat GF, Diech GS, Wynder EL: Bladder cancer in nonsmokers. Cancer 1986 (57):362-367
142 Rebelakos A, Trichopoulos E, Tzonouo A et al: Tobacco smoking, coffee drinking, and occupation as risk factors for bladder cancer in Greece. JNCI 1985 (75):455-461
143 Marrett LD, Walter SD, Meigs JW: Coffee drinking and bladder cancer in Connecticut. Am J Epidemiol 1983 (117):113-122

144 Hartge P, Hoover R, West DW et al: Coffee drinking and risk of bladder cancer. JNCI 1983 (70):1021-1026
145 Binstock M, Krakow D, Stamler J et al: Coffee and pancreatic cancer: an analysis of international mortality data. Am J Epidemiol 1983 (118):680-684
146 Whittemore AS, Paffenbarger RS, Anderson K et al: Early precursors of pancreatic cancer in college men. J Chron Dis 1983 (36):251-256
147 Heuch I, Kvale G, Jacobsen BK et al: Use of alcohol, tobacco and coffee. Br J Cancer 1983 (48):637-643
148 MacMahon B, Yen S, Trichopoulos D et al: Coffee and cancer of the pancreas. N Eng J Med 1981 (304):630-633
149 Hsieh C, MacMahon B, Yen S et al: Coffee and pancreatic cancer, chapter 2. N Eng J Med 1986 (315):584-588
150 Gold LN, Gordis L, Diener MD et al: Diet and other risk factors for cancer of the pancreas. Cancer 1985 (55):460-467
151 Mack TM, Yu MC, Hanisch R et al: Pancreas cancer and smoking, beverage consumption, and past medical history. JNCI 1986 (74):569-573
152 Norrell SE, Ahlbom A, Erwald R et al: Diet and pancreatic cancer: a case-control study. Am J Epidemiol 1986 (124):894-902
153 Wynder EL, Hall NE, Polansky M: Epidemiology of coffee and pancreatic cancer. Cancer Res 1983 (43):3300-3306
154 Lubin F, Ron E, Wax Y: Coffee and methylxanthines and breast cancer: A case-control study. JNCI 1985 (74):569-573
155 Rosenberg L, Miller DR, Helmrich SP et al: Breast cancer and the consumption of coffee. Am J Epidemiol 1980 (122):391-399
156 Le MG: Coffee consumption, benign breast disease, and breast cancer (Letter to the editor). Am J Epidemiol 1985 (122):721
157 La Vecchia CS, Franceschi S, Decarli A et al: Coffee drinking and risk of epithelial overian cancer. Int J Cancer 1984 (33):559-562
158 Trichopoulos D, Papapostolou M, Polychronopoulou A: Coffee and ovarian cancer. Int J Cancer 1981 (28):691-693
159 Byers T, Marshall J, Graham S et al: A case-control study of dietary and nondietary factors in ovarian cancer. JNCI 1983 (71):681-686
160 Miller DR, Rosenberg L, Kaufman DL et al: Epithelial ovarian cancer and coffee drinking. Int J Epidemiol 1987 (16):13-17
161 Heilbrun LK, Nomura A, Stemmermann GN: Black tea consumption and cancer risk: A prospective study. Br J Cancer 1986 (54):677-683
162 Kinlen LJ, McPherson K: Pancreas cancer and coffee and tea consumption. A case control study. Br J Cancer 1984 (49):93
163 Miller CT, Neutel CI, Nair RC et al: Relative importance of risk factors in bladder carcinogenesis. J Chron Dis 1978 (31):51-56
164 Morgan RW, Jain MG: Bladder cancer: Smoking, beverages and artificial sweeteners. Can Med Assoc J 1974 (111):1067-1070
165 Sullivan JW: Epidemiologic survey of bladder cancer in greater New Orleans. J Urol 1982 (128):281-283
166 Stocks P: Cancer mortality in relation to national consumption of cigarettes, solid food, tea and coffee. Br J Cancer 1970 (24):215
167 Phillips RL, Snowdon DA: Dietary relationship with fatal colorectal cancer among Seventh-Day Adventists. JNCI 1985 (74):307
168 Tajima A, Tominaga S: Dietary habits and gastrointestinal cancers: a comparative case-control study of stomach and large intestinal cancers in Nagoya, Japan. Jap J Cancer Res 1985 (76):705
169 Burbank F, Fraumeni JF: Synthetic sweetener consumption and bladder cancer trends in the United States. Nature 1970 (227):296-297
170 Armstrong B, Doll R: Bladder cancer mortality in England and Wales in relation to cigarette smoking and saccharin consumption. Br J Prev Soc Med 1974 (28):233-240
171 Kessler II: Cancer Mortality among diabetics. JNCI 1970 (44):673-686
172 Kessler II: Non-nutritive sweeteners and human bladder cancer. Preliminary findings. J Urol 1976 (115):143-146
173 Kessler II, Clark JP: Saccharin, cyclamate, and human bladder cancer: no evidence of an association. J Am Med Assoc 1978 (240):349-355
174 Howe GR, Burch JD, Miller AB et al: Artificial sweeteners and human bladder cancer. Lancet 1977 (2):578-581
175 Hoover RN, Strasser P: Artificial sweeteners in human bladder cancer. Preliminary results. Lancet 1980 (91):837-840
176 Cartwright RA, Adib R, Glashan R, Gray BK: The epidemiology of bladder cancer in West Yorkshire. A preliminary report on non-occupational aetiologies. Carcinogenesis 1981 (2):343-347
177 Jensen OM, Knudsen JB, Sorensen BL et al: Artificial sweeteners and absence of bladder risk in Copenhagen. Int J Cancer 1983 (32):577-582
178 Morrison AS, Buring JE: Artificial sweeteners and cancer of the lower urinary tract. N Eng J Med 1980 (302):537-541
179 Morrison AS, Verhoek WG, Leck I et al: Artificial sweeteners and bladder cancer in Manchester, U.K. and Nagoya, Japan. Br J Cancer 1982 (45):332-336
180 Najem GR, Louris DB, Seebode JJ et al: Lifetime occupation, smoking, caffeine, saccharin, hair dyes, and bladder carcinogenesis. Int J Epidemiol 1982 (11):212-217
181 Wynder EL, Stellman SD: Artificial sweetener use and bladder cancer: a case control study. Science 1980 (207):1214-1216
182 National Research Council. The Health Effects of Nitrate, Nitrite, and N-Nitroso Compounds-Part I of a 2-Part Study. Washington, DC: National Academy Press 1981
183 Magee PN, Barnes JM: Carcinogenic nitroso compounds. Adv Cancer Res 1967 (10):163-246
184 Rao TK, Lijinsky W, Epler JL (eds) Genotoxicology of N-nitroso Compounds. New York: Plenum Press 1984

185 Lijinsky W: The significance of N-nitroso compounds as environmental carcinogens. J Env Sci Health 1986 (C4):1-45
186 Armijo R, Coulson AH: Epidemiology of stomach cancer in Chile - The role of nitrogen fertilizers. Int J Epidemiol 1975 (4):301-309
187 Armijo R, Gonzalez A, Orellana M et al: Epidemology of gastric cancer in Chile. II. Nitrate exposures and stomach cancer frequency. Int J Epidemiol 1981 (10):57-62
188 Cuello C, Correa P, Haenszel W et al: Gastric cancer in Columbia. I. Cancer risk and suspect environmental agents. JNCI 1976 (57):1015-1020
189 Haenszel W, Kurihara M, Segi M, Lee RKC: Stomach cancer among Japanese in Hawaii. JNCI 1972 (49):969-988
190 Wynder EL, Onderdonk J, Mantel N: An epidemiology investigation of cancer of the bladder. Cancer 1963 (16):1388-1407
191 Radomski JL, Greenwald D, Hearn WL et al: Nitrosamine formation in the bladder infections and its role in the etiology of bladder cancer. J Urol 1978 (120):48-58
192 Yang CS: Research on esophageal cancer in China. Cancer Res 1980 (40):2633-2644
193 Lu SH, Montesano R, Zhang MW et al: Relevance of N-nitrosamines to esophageal cancer in China. J Clin Physiol 1986 (4):51-58
194 Choi NW, Entwistle DW, Michaluk W: Gastric cancer in Icelanders in Manitoba. Isr J Med Sci (7):1500-1508
195 Kriebel D, Jowett D: Stomach cancer mortality in the north central states - high risk is not limited to the foreign-born. Nutr Cancer 1979 (1):8-12
196 Lijinsky W, Shubik P: Benzo[a]pyrene and other polynuclear hydrocarbons in charcoal-broiled meat. Science 1964 (145):53-55
197 Correa P, Fontham E, Pickle LW et al: Dietary determinants of gastric cancer in South Louisiana inhabitants. JNCI 1985 (75):645-654
198 Linsell CA, Peers FG: Aflatoxin and liver cell cancer. Trans R Soc Trop Med Hyg 1977 (71):471-473
199 Oettle AG: The etiology of primary carcinoma of the liver in Africa: A critical appraisal of previous ideas with an outline of the mycotoxin hypothesis. S Afr Med J 1965 (39):817-825
200 Keen P, Martin P: The toxicity and fungal infestation of food-stuffs in Swaziland in relation to harvesting and storage. Trop Geogr Med 1971 (23):35-43
201 Alpert ME, Hutt MSR, Wogan GN, Davidson CS: Association between aflatoxin content of food and hepatoma frequency in Uganda. Cancer 1971 (28):253-260
202 Peers FG, Gilman GA, Linsell CA: Dietary aflatoxins and human liver cancer: A study in Swaziland. Int J Cancer 1976 (17):167-176
203 Peers F, Bosch X, Kaldor J et al: Aflatoxin exposure, hepatitus B virus infection and liver cancer in Swaziland. Int J Cancer 1987 (150):545-553
204 Peers FG, Linsell CA: Dietary aflatoxins and liver cancer. A population-based study in Kenya. Br J Cancer 1973 (27):473-484
205 van Rensburg SJ, van der Watt, Purchase IFH et al: Primary liver cancer rate and aflatoxin intake in a high cancer area. S Afr Med J 1974 (48):2508a-2508d
206 van Rensburg SJ, Cook-Mozaffari P, Van Schalkwyk DJ et al: Hepatocellular carcinoma and dietary aflatoxin in Mozambique and Transkei. Br J Cancer 1985 (51):713-726
207 Shank RC, Bhamarapravati N, Gordon JE, Wogan GN: Dietary aflatoxins and human liver cancer. IV. Incidence of primary liver cancer in the municipal populations of Thailand. Food Cosmet Toxicol 1972 (10):171-179
208 Shank RC, Gordan JE, Wogan GN et al: Dietary aflatoxins and human liver cancer. III. Field survey or rural Thai families for ingested aflatoxins. Food Cosmet Toxicol 1972 (10):71-84
209 Wogan GN: Dietary factors and special epidemiological situations of liver cancer in Thailand and Africa. Cancer Res 1975 (35):3499-3502
210 Armstrong B: The epidemiology of cancer in the People's Republic of China. Int J Epidemiol 1980 (9):305-315
211 Tung TC, Ling K.H: Study on aflatoxin of food stuffs in Taiwan. Vitaminol J 1968 (14 Suppl):48-52
212 Yen FS, Shen KN: Epidemiology and early diagnosis of primary liver cancer in China. Adv Cancer Res 1986 (47):297-329
213 Bulatao-Jame J, Almero EM, Castro MC et al: A case-control study of primary liver cancer risk from aflatoxin exposure. Int J Epidemiol 1982 (11):112-119
214 Ayoola EA: Synergism between hepatitis B virus and aflatoxin in hepatocellular carcinoma. IARC Sci Publ 1984 (63):167-179
215 Beasley RP, Hwang L, Lin C et al: Hepatocellular carcinoma and hepatitis B virus. Lancet 1981 (2):1129-1133
216 Chien MC, Tong MJ, Lo KJ et al: Hepatitis B viral markers in patients with primary hepatocellular carcinoma in Taiwan. JNCI 1981 (66):475-479
217 Prince AN, Szumess W, Michon J et al: A case-control study of the association between primary liver cancer and hepatitis B infection in Senegal. Int J Cancer 1975 (16):376-383
218 Stora C, Dvorackova I: Aflatoxin viral hepatitis and primary liver cancer. J Med Clin Exp Theor 1987 (18):23-41
219 Sun T, Chu J: Carcinogenesis and prevention strategy of liver cancer in areas differing in prevalence. J Cell Physiol 1984 (3 Suppl):39-44
220 Yeh FS, Mo CC, Yen RC: Risk factors for hepatocellular carcinoma in Guangxi Peoples Republic of China. NCI Monogr 1985 (69):47-48

Methodological Issues in the Investigation of Diet and Cancer in Humans

Elio Riboli

Unit of Analytical Epidemiology, International Agency for Research on Cancer, 69372 Lyon Cédex , France

Introduction

Interest in the relation between diet and cancer has grown in recent years from the points of view of both scientific research and public health action.

The rational support for such a large public concern is that if elements of diet are related to cancer aetiology, their impact in terms of attributable risk could be very large because of the high proportion of people potentially exposed (even if the relative increase in cancer risk is moderate), and the corresponding preventable fraction would in theory be proportionally large.

All three major attempts to define the proportion of all cancer cases/deaths due to identified and less well-defined causes [1,2,3] agree in attributing a conspicuous role to dietary factors; Wynder and Gori attributed 40% and 57% of all cancer cases in males and females, respectively, to dietary factors, while Higginson and Muir attributed 30% in males and 63% in females of all cancer cases to life-style factors, among which diet was predominant. Doll and Peto have provided a "best estimate" of the proportion of all cancers that could be attributed to diet of 35%, which could range from a minimum of 10% to a maximum of 70%. The most relevant aspect of this estimate is probably not the central figure of 35% (although it was carefully derived from the available scientific evidence) but the width of the "range of acceptable estimates".

A large interval to an estimated attributable risk is sometimes due to a lack of reliable data on the proportion of people among the general population exposed to a well recognised carcinogen, as often occurs with chemicals used in a variety of industrial processes. This does not seem the main reason for the uncertainty surrounding the estimates of the AR for diet, for which figures at the population levels of the distribution of subjects according to their consumption of main items of food and nutrients are available for several countries. Although such figures derived from nutritional surveys are not always representative of the general population, they are of much higher quality than that which is available for many recognised carcinogens (e.g. occupational chemicals).

The main cause of the uncertainty still surrounding the aetiological role of specific elements of human diet is that in many cases the scientific evidence in humans is still limited. For several cancers, the results from a fairly large number of epidemiological studies are available, thus it is not a lack of data, but rather a lack of fully convincing data on humans, which explains the residual doubts.

Major Problems of Studies on Diet and Cancer in Humans

Modern epidemiology has adequate tools to pick up the association between cancer, or other chronic diseases, and a given aetiological agent, particularly when the risk for those exposed relative to those non-exposed is rather high (even if the exposure is assessed with some approximation) or when the exposure can be measured with good validity and precision (even if the associated risk is low).

Table 1. Correlation coefficients between intake of selected nutrients from different epidemiological studies

	Sex	No. of subjects	Vitamin C, beta-carotene	Vitamin C, fibre	Beta-carotene, fibre	Saturated fat, protein
Ontario, Canada	M	832	-	0.49	-	0.77
[27]	F	787	-	0.54	-	0.75
Marseilles, France [28]	M+F	399	-	0.85	-	0.78
Varese, Italy	M	487	0.46	0.67	0.46	0.71
	F	503	0.47	0.67	0.50	0.70
Pamplona, Spain	M	420	0.43	0.42	0.33	0.72
	F	135	0.67	0.52	0.43	0.74
Calvados, France	M	922	0.61	0.73	0.52	0.67
[19] *	F	1053	0.65	0.76	0.55	0.68

* Above figures not shown in paper referred to, but calculated from the data of the study

Typical examples of the first case are the studies on tobacco, heavy alcohol intake and several industrial carcinogens, while the recent NCI-IARC collaborative study [4] on low level radiation exposure and second primary cancer in women treated with radium for cervical cancer is a good example of the second.

Studies on diet and cancer in human subjects do not generally fall in either of the two previous cases. From what we know today, it seems that we face the difficulty of investigating an exposure (diet) for which it is quite difficult to have good measurements and at the same time the associated relative risks are expected to be moderately low.

Three major problems need to be solved in order to improve the explanatory power of investigation on diet and cancer in humans:

1) The information on dietary habits covered by virtually all the published studies refers to a limited period of life. In case-control studies it usually refers to diet during approx. 2 years preceding diagnosis in cases and to an equivalent period in controls. In the few long-term prospective studies carried out on diet and cancer the information on diet was collected only once, at the time preceding the subjects' enrolment without additional information on changes which may have occurred during the follow-up period.

2) Individual diet is usually a very complex mixture with important day to day variations. The number of chemical compounds ingested with food and drink is very large and it is difficult to obtain adequate information to estimate the intake and eventually distinguish the health effects of specific substances.

This is due in part to methodological limitations of dietary assessment methods, some of which, although of practical use in large epidemiological studies, provide information of limited quality on food chemical composition. On the other hand, methods based on chemical analyses of duplicate portions of the food actually eaten by the subjects under study are so elaborate and expensive that they have not been applied so far in large epidemiological studies.

An additional problem is that some nutrients tend to "go together" as they are eaten in combination or are ingredients of the same dishes or components of the same food. For instance, it has often been found that subjects with high intake of vitamin C tend also to have high intake of beta-carotene because these two micronutrients are often provided by the same fruits and vegetables.

Table 1 provides as an example the correlations at the individual level found in different studies between intake of vitamin C and beta-carotene, vitamin C and fibre, beta-carotene and fibre, saturated fat and protein.

3) The risk associated with any specific food item is likely to be low both in terms of relative and attributable risk, notwithstanding some remarkable exceptions, such as the very high risk of laryngeal, pharyngeal and oesophageal cancer, due to elevated life-long alcohol consumption [5], or the reported association between Cantonese salted fish and nasopharyngeal cancer in South-East Asia [6].

This does not deny the fact that dietary habits could be responsible for a substantial increase in the risk of some cancers, but it stresses the need for evaluating diet as a whole, taking into account all major energy-providing components (fat, carbohydrates, proteins and alcohol) as well as non energy-providing substances (vitamins, mineral salts, contaminants).

Estimation of Individual Diet: Current Limitations and Future Perspectives

Dietary Assessment Methods

Several instruments have been proposed for the estimation of individual diet based on the subject's recall of recent diet (e.g. recall of preceding 1-3 days) or recall of usual diet over a longer period (e.g. 1 year) or on prospective recording of the food actually eaten over a few days (e.g. 3-7 day diet diary). These methods have been described in detail in comprehensive reviews [7,8]. More recently, several variants of the traditional approaches have been tested to estimate their relative validity and repeatability in methodological studies [9-19].

Some of the proposed methods allow simple estimation of the usual intake of a limited number of food groups in terms of weekly frequency, while others provide enough information to compute the average daily intake of specific nutrients. The latter types of dietary methods are more informative in studies on diet and cancer.

In several methodological studies the reference method was a diet diary, with food amounts estimated by weighing, which described the subject's diet over several days or weeks.

The correlations between the estimates of nutrient intake provided by the reference method and by alternative methods (e.g. food frequency, dietary history) range at best in the order of 0.5 to 0.7. This level of concordance between what is still considered the "gold standard" of all dietary methods (2-4 weeks of weighed diet diary) and the methods actually used in epidemiological studies can be considered an acceptable compromise between desirable quality and practical feasibility in large studies. On the other hand, a correlation in the order of 0.5 and 0.7 between the "truth" and its empirical measurement may lead to serious underestimation of any real association between cancer and diet.

In addition, there are several dietary methods developed for use in epidemiological studies which aim at estimating intake of one or just a few nutrients (e.g. vitamin A or C, fat). The rationale for these methods is that they should allow a careful estimation of the nutrient which is being investigated without wasting time and effort to obtain data on all nutrients. This reasoning may sound appealing and to a certain extent can turn out to be useful. This approach becomes debatable when the method allows no estimate at all for the intake of major energy-providing nutrients (protein, fat, carbohydrates and alcohol) and of caloric intake itself. In this case it becomes impossible in data analysis to explore whether a putative protective or causal association with a particular nutrient may be due to confounding by other components of diet.

The process of estimating nutrient intake is quite complex and it deserves to be briefly considered in order to fully appreciate the present difficulties and establish in which direction scientific research should be developed.

The fundamental steps involved in the estimation of individual nutrient intake will be schematically illustrated, taking as an example the most complete and accurate dietary methods actually used in cancer epidemiology (dietary history or food frequency with estimation of food portion size) which allow the computation of nutrient intake (Fig. 1).

The goal of the whole process is to estimate, in terms of nutrient intake, the real individual diet. The first ingredient is the Dietary Assessment Method which provides, once the information has been collected, a "vector" of the amount of food consumed per unit of time. This vector is then multiplied by the matrix (food x nutrients) usually called the Food Composition Table. The amount of a specific nutrient is then summed over all foods containing it (according to the content given in the food table). The result is a "vector" con-

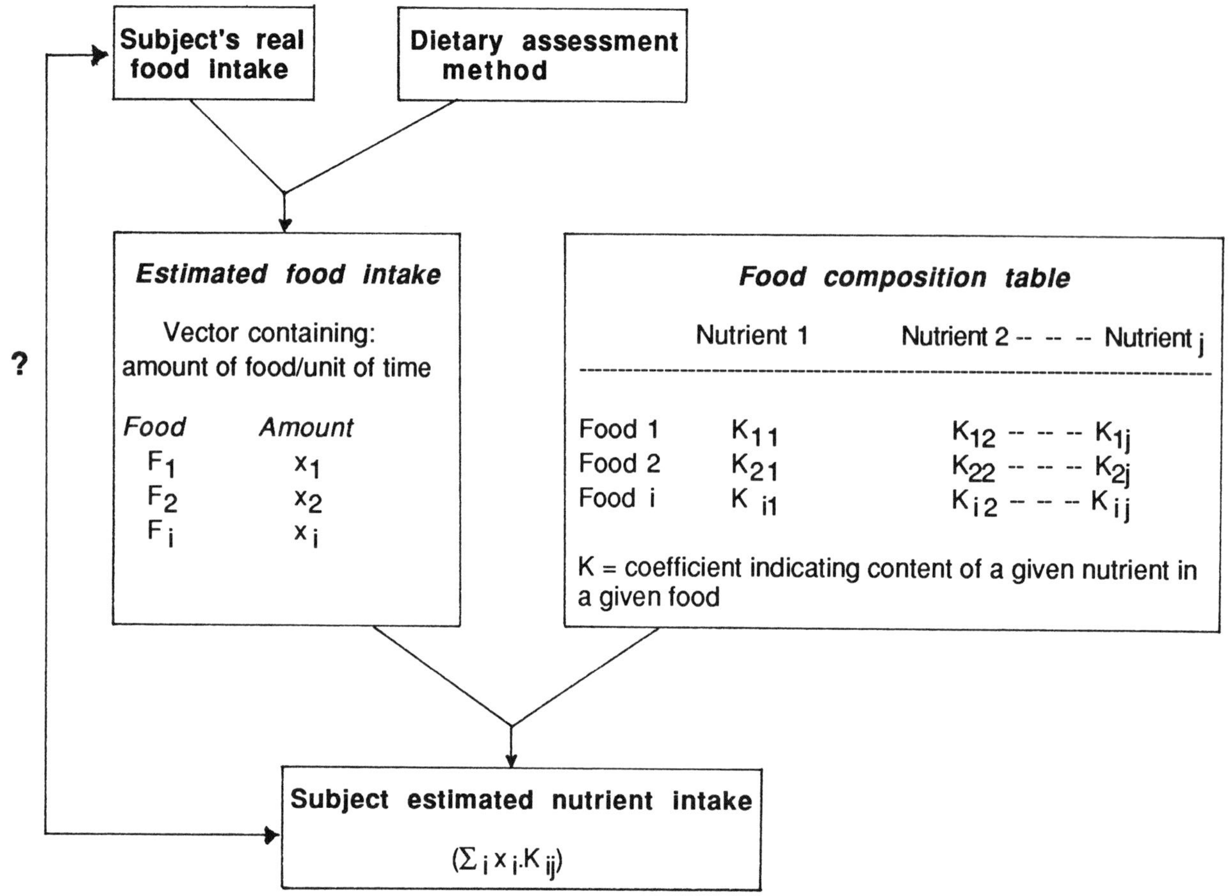

Fig. 1. Scheme of the process of estimating nutrient intake by means of dietary methods and food composition tables

taining the estimated nutrient intake in a given standard time period. The extent to which the final result will be a close description of the real individual intake depends not only on the dietary method as discussed above but also on the food tables. The coefficient of nutrient content of specific foods is at best an approximation of the real content of the food consumed by the subject in a given year.

Considering, for example, the vitamin C content of potato, the first approximation derives from the fact that the value in the food table is usually the average vitamin C content found by repeated chemical analyses on different types of potatoes, possibly during different periods of the year.

The second approximation is that this particular value may or may not be relevant for the potatoes available on the market and consumed by the subjects during the study period. For example, the vitamin C content in potato decreases with time from the harvest and varies with the type of cooking.

A third approximation is that several food items sharing some similarities are quite commonly pooled in a unique food group because the subjects under study would not be able to provide the details of their consumption separately for each item. For example, beef meat may be an important source of total fat intake but the fat content of beef varies from 5% for silverside to about 30% for foreribs [20]. The real amount of fat provided by beef for a given subject may in fact be quite different from what could be estimated with standard food tables where a unique average fat content is provided for any cut of beef. In addition to these problems, it should be added that food composition varies over time and from one region to another, due to changes in food technology, while the food composition table is at best available at the national level and is (with few exceptions) not very often updated. In fact it should be emphasised that food tables based on chemical measurements of food samples are only available for a few countries in the world and that for several European countries national food tables based on measurement of local foods are not yet available.

Biological Markers of Diet

Several laboratory techniques have been developed in the field of human nutrition to investigate nutritional status, dietary intake and metabolic functions. Many of these techniques are very accurate but unfortunately their use requires quite sophisticated procedures and at present cannot be exploited outside a specialised nutritional ward. There are, nevertheless, some biochemical investigations which require relatively simple approaches, at least during the phase of the procedure involving the direct participation of the subjects under study [21].

In recent years interest in biochemical markers of diet was also stimulated by the recognition of the limitations of current dietary assessment methods. Some biological markers have already been used in the early prospective studies on diet and cardiovascular diseases conducted in the 1950s and 60s. These were chiefly the cholesterol and lipid concentrations in blood.

In diet and cancer epidemiology the use of biological markers has so far been very limited. With the exception of a few studies on vitamin A and E, selenium and cholesterol, most of the published investigations were simply based on the information provided by dietary questionnaires.

Table 2 provides a non-exhaustive list of markers which have been proposed for use in nutritional epidemiology.

Measures of energy expenditure, energy balance and metabolic rate have been omitted on purpose because, although a number of simplified and miniaturised devices have been proposed, their cost and complexity prevent their use in the field conditions of current epidemiological studies. Measures of carbohydrate intake, on the contrary, are not mentioned simply because there is not a single method available yet.

Table 2. Biological markers of dietary intake which have been considered for use in nutritional epidemiology

Marker of:	Marker
Protein	24-hour urinary nitrogen
	24-hour 3-methylhistidine
Fat	Fatty acids in:
	adipose tissue
	erythrocytes
	cheek cells
	plasma lipids
Vitamin	Retinol in plasma
	Carotenoids in plasma
	Ascorbic acid in:
	plasma
	leucocytes
	saliva
	Lingual ascorbic acid test
	Alpha-tocopherol in:
	plasma
Mineral salt	Selenium in:
	plasma
	erythrocytes
	nails, hair
	24-hour urine
	glutathion peroxidase activity
	Zinc in:
	plasma
	saliva
	24-hour urine
	hair

Of particular interest to the investigation of the relation between diet and cancer are markers of fat intake. Although good quantitative markers of total fat intake are not available, a number of methods have been developed to evaluate the qualitative characteristics of fat intake. All these methods are based on the analyses of the fatty acid composition of either depot fat or membrane structural lipids from cell samples of the human body.

Analyses of triglyceride fatty acids in depot fat was proposed as a method to investigate the relative proportion of fatty acids in diet almost 30 years ago [22]. It requires a small sample of subcutaneous adipose tissue which is usually taken by a special needle (1.5 mm diameter) [23] or with a skin biopsy punch (33 mm diameter) [24].

The method relies on the fact that the turnover of fatty acids in adipose tissue is very slow and for subjects whose body weight remains stable, the half-life of fatty acids is in the order of 600 days [25]. The method, therefore, provides a picture of the type of fat consumed during the previous 2 or 3 years.

Subcutaneous fat biopsy has not been widely used so far, mainly because the sampling procedure is believed to be painful and not acceptable by study subjects. Recent experiences tend to indicate that the method is quite acceptable and does not cause any major discomfort, at least no more than a common venipuncture [23].

Other qualitative methods proposed for the study of fat intake are the analyses of phospholipid fatty acids from cell membranes (adipocytes, platelet, cheek cell and erythrocytes) and fatty acids in plasma.

Fatty acids enter into the composition of cell membranes as a component of complex phospholipid molecules [26]. The fatty acid composition varies according to the type of cell for a given subject and it reflects the dietary intake during a period roughly corresponding to the half-life of the cells.

Table 3 provides some indications of the composition of major fatty acids of depot fat, cell membranes and plasma provided by various studies [21].

The values shown indicate that the picture provided by different specimens is very different; therefore, the composition of fatty acids from any of these methods can be related to dietary intake only in relative rather than in absolute terms. For example, the linoleic acid percentage of total fatty acids is highest in plasma (around 30%) and lowest in platelet membranes (about 5-7%), with intermediate levels in depot fat and adipocyte membranes. On the other hand, oleic acid usually accounts for more than 45% of total depot fat while its concentration in plasma is about 20% of total fatty acids [21].

Table 3. Percent composition of major fatty acids of depot fat, cell membranes and plasma, derived from various studies

	Adipose tissue - depot fat				Adipocyte membranes	Platelet membranes		Cheek cell membranes	Erythro-cyte	Plasma 1)
	Wood et al. [29]	Field et al. [30]	Berry et al. [31]	v.Staveren et al. [32]	Field et al. [30]	Wood et al. [29]	Renaud et al. [33]	McMurchie et al. [34]	Angelico et al. [35]	
Saturated										
Myristic (14:0)	4.0	3.0	2.4	2.8	-	0.2	-	-	2.7	-
Palmitic (16:0)	23.4	18.8	19.2	17.9	23.3	15.6	13.2-14.3	23.4	25.5	20-23
Stearic (18:0)	5.0	3.3	3.7	3.5	11.2	19.9	17.5-18.2	20.4	11.9	
Monounsaturated										
Palmitoleic (16:1)	8.8	6.3	6.5	7.7	4.9	1.0	-	6.7	4.5	-
Oleic (18:1)	44.0	49.7	46.1	43.7	13.7	19.1	15.0-17.3	37.1	17.2	19-25
Polyunsaturated										
Linolenic (18:2)	8.9	13.1	16.3	14.2	13.9	5.1	5.6-7.0	8.4	8.3	27-34
Linolenic (18:3)	3.0	0.6	1.9	0.9	3.5	1.6	-	-	1.2	0.2-0.8
Arachidonic (20:4)	0.6	0.2	-	-	4.2	28.0	26.8-29.5	3.8	6.7	6-9
Other polyunsaturated	-	-	-	-	8.4	-	6.1-6.7	-	7.1	-
P/S	-	0.57	0.73	0.72	0.83	1.17	≈ 1.0	0.28	0.77	

1) Range of values derived from several reports in medical literature and physiology textbooks

Conclusions

In conclusion, it can be said that, on the one hand, there is not a unique and best dietary assessment method that can be recommended for all epidemiological studies; on the other hand, there are some good rules which should be taken into consideration when planning new research, and which can be summarised as follows:

1. Use a dietary assessment method able to provide information on total energy intake as well as on major nutrients, even if the focus of the study is on a particular nutrient.
2. Adapt the method to local culture and local eating habits, such as eating pattern during the day, use of local casseroles and recipes.
3. Adapt the dietary assessment method to the educational level of the subjects to be investigated. For example, self-administered questionnaires can substantially reduce the study cost but require that the subjects be able to read correctly, understand the questions, estimate frequency and amount of their food consumption, write the correct answers. Questionnaires administered by an interviewer are more expensive but less dependent on the subjects' education.
4. Test the repeatability and relative validity of the proposed method under field conditions. Demonstration of repeatability (reliability) requires that the instrument be administered to the same subjects 2 or 3 times within a convenient time period. Relative validity can be demonstrated by comparing it with an appropriate standard such as a more sophisticated method and/or a set of biochemical markers of diet.
5. Adapt Food Composition Tables to food locally consumed. Data on food composition may sometimes be available locally from institutions in charge of food analyses for administrative or health surveillance purposes. In addition, the breakdown or the pooling of food groups (in the Food Table) should be adapted to local dietary habits.
6. Biochemical markers of nutrient intake should be used when appropriate and feasible to complement the information provided by other methods.
7. Markers of individual genetic traits may enable researchers to identify subgroups of subjects more or less susceptible to the health effects of particular dietary habits (e.g. differences in cholesterol metabolism, inherited risk of colon cancer, etc.).
8. Repeated measurements on the same subjects may be considered if the precision of a dietary assessment method or a biological marker is not satisfactory when based on a unique measurement because of biological day to day variations and/or random error of the method. Double sources providing independent information (e.g. spouse or other members of the family) can improve the validity of the information on individual diet.

REFERENCES

1 Wynder EL, Gori GB: Contribution of the environment to cancer incidence: an epidemiologic exercise. JNCI 1977 (58):825-832

2 Higginson J, Muir CS: Environmental carcinogenesis: misconceptions and limitations to cancer control. JNCI 1979 (63):1291-1298

3 Peto R, Doll R, Buckley JD, Sporn MB: Can dietary beta-carotene materially reduce human cancer rates? Nature 1981 (290):201-208

4 Boice JD Jr, Blettner M, Kleinerman RA et al: Radiation dose and leukemia risk in patients treated for cancer of the cervix. JNCI 1987 (79):1295-1311

5 IARC Monographs on the Evaluation of the Carcinogenic Risk of Chemicals to Humans: Alcohols and Alcoholic Beverages. Lyon 1988, Vol 44 (in press)

6 Yu MC, Ho JH, Henderson BE, Armstrong RW: Epidemiology of nasopharyngeal carcinoma in Malaysia and Hong-Kong. NCI Monogr 1985 (69):203-207

7 Marr J: Individual dietary surveys: purposes and methods. World Rev Nutr Diet 1971 (13):105-164

8 Block G: A review of validations of dietary assessment methods. Am J Epidemiol 1982 (115):492-505

9 Jain MG, Harrison L, Howe GR, Miller AB: Evaluation of a self-administered dietary questionnaire for use in a cohort study. Am J Clin Nutr 1982 (36):931-935

10 Bazzarre TL, Yuhas JA: Comparative evaluation of methods of collecting food intake data for cancer epidemiology studies. Nutr Cancer 1983 (5):201-214

11 Byers TE, Rosenthal RI, Marshall JR, Rzepka TF, Cummings KM, Graham S: Dietary history from the distant past: a methodological study. Nutr Cancer 1983 (5):69-77

12 van Leeuwen FE, de Vet HCW, Hayes RB, van Staveren WA, West CE, Hautvast JGAJ: An assessment of the relative validity of retrospective interviewing for measuring dietary intake. Am J Epidemiol 1983 (118):752-758

13 Chu SY, Kolonel LN, Hankin JH, Lee J: A comparison of frequency and quantitative dietary methods for epidemiologic studies of diet and disease. Am J Epidemiol 1984 (119):323-334

14 Humble CG, Samet JM, Skipper BE: Comparison of self- and surrogate-reported dietary information. Am J Epidemiol 1984 (119):86-98

15 Möller-Jensen O, Wahrendorf J, Rosenqvist A, Geser A: The reliability of questionnaire-derived dietary information and temporal stability of food habits in individuals. Am J Epidemiol 1984 (120):281-290

16 Muller BJ, Krantzler NJ, Grivetti LE, Schutz HG, Meiselman HL: Validity of a food frequency questionnaire for determination of individual food intake. Am J Clin Nutr 1984 (39):136-143

17 Willett WC, Sampson L, Stampfer MJ, Rosner B, Bain C, Sitschi J, Hennekens CH, Speizer FE: Reproducibility and validity of a semiquantitative food frequency questionnaire. Am J Epidemiol 1985 (122):51-65

18 Riboli E, Caperle M, Sabatino C, Crespi M: Evaluation of dietary assessment methods: pilot phase of a case-control study on colorectal polyps. It J Gastr 1986 (18):245-248

19 Riboli E, Péquignot G, Repetto F, Axerio M, Faymond L, Boffetta P, Zubiri A, Del Moral A. Estève J, Tuyns AJ: A comparative study of smoking, drinking and dietary habits in population samples in Italy, Spain, Switzerland and France. I. Study design and dietary habits. Rev Epidémiol Santé Publ 1987 (in press)

20 Paul AA, Southgate DAT: McCance and Widdowson's The Composition of Foods, 4th Edition. London: Her Majesty's Stationery Office, 1978

21 Riboli E, Röhnholm H, Saracci R: Biological markers of diet. Cancer Surv 1987 (6):685-718

22 Hirsch J, Farquhar JW, Ahrens EH, Peterson ML, Stoffel W: Studies of adipose tissue in man: a microtechnic for sampling and analysis. Am J Clin Nutr 1960 (8):499-511

23 Beynen AC, Katan MB: Rapid sampling and long-term storage of subcutaneous adipose-tissue biopsies for determination of fatty acid composition. Am J Clin Nutr 1985 (42):317-322

24 Smith WCS, Tavendale R, Tunstall-Pedoe H: Simplified subcutaneous fat biopsy for nutritional surveys. Human Nutr: Clin Nutr 1986 (40C):323-325

25 Beynen AC, Hermus RJJ, Hautvast JGAJ: A mathematical relationship between the fatty acid composition of the diet and that of the adipose tissue in man. Am J Clin Nutr 1980 (33):81-85

26 Ways P, Hanahan DJ: Characterization and qualification of red cell lipids in normal men. J Lip Res 1964 (5):318-328

27 Jain M, Cook GM, Davis FG et al: A case-control study of diet and colo-rectal cancer. Int J Cancer 1980 (26):757-768

28 Macquart-Moulin G, Riboli E, Cornee J et al: Case-control study on colorectal cancer and diet in Marseilles. Int J Cancer 1986 (38):183-191

29 Wood DA, Butler S, Riemersma R, Thomson M, Oliver MF: Adipose tissue and platelet fatty acids and coronary heart disease in Scottish men. Lancet 1984 (ii):117-121

30 Field CJ, Angel A, Clandinin MT: Relationship of diet to the fatty acid composition of human adipose tissue structural and stored lipids. Am J Clin Nutr 1985 (42):1206-1220

31 Berry EM, Hirsch J, Most J, McNamara DJ, Thornton J: The relationship of dietary fat to plasma lipid levels as studied by factor analysis of adipose tissue fatty acid composition in a free-living population of middle-aged American men. Am J Clin Nutr 1986 (44):220-231

32 van Staveren WJ, Deurenberg P, Katan MB, Burema J, de Groot ICPGM, Hoffmans MDAF: Validity of the fatty acid composition of subcutaneous fat tissue microbiopsies as an estimate of the long-term average fatty acid composition of the diet to separate individuals. Am J Epidemiol 1986 (123):455-463

33 Renaud S, Fodsey E, Dumont E, Thevenon C, Ortchanian E, Martin JL: Influence of long-term diet modification on platelet function and composition in Moselle farmers. Am J Clin Nutr 1986 (43):136-150

34 McMurchie EJ, Margetts BM, Beilin LJ, Croft KD, Vandongen R, Armstrong BK: Dietary-induced changes in the fatty acid composition of human cheek cell phospholipids: correlation with changes in the dietary polyunsaturated/saturated fat ratio. Am J Clin Nutr 1984 (39):975-980

35 Angelico F, Amedeo P, Guccione P, Montali A, Menotti A, Ricci G, Urbinati GC: Dietary and red blood cell fatty acid changes after a four-year dietary intervention in the Rome project of Coronary Heart Disease Prevention. Clin Ter Cardiovasc 1982 (1):1-7

Alcohol

O.M. Jensen [1] and A.B. Miller [2]

1) Danish Cancer Registry, Institute of Cancer Epidemiology of the Danish Cancer Society, Landskronagade 66, DK-2100 Copenhagen, Denmark

2) Department of Preventive Medicine and Biostatistics, University of Toronto, Toronto, Ontario, M5S 1A8, Canada

Introduction

Associations between alcohol drinking and certain types of cancer have been observed for many years. Because some of the associations vary by site, the evidence will be considered in relation to individual cancer sites.

Tobacco-Associated Cancers

Oral cavity and pharynx

Increased mortality from oropharyngeal cancer was observed among persons in occupations involving high alcohol consumption, as well as among alcoholics, whereas alcohol abstainers such as Seventh-Day Adventists and Mormons in the U.S. have decreased risks [1-3]. In a cohort study of 14,000 Danish brewery workers who were not alcoholics, but had an above average consumption of beer, the incidence of pharyngeal cancer was twice as high as general population rates [4].

A study of 543 men with cancer of the lip, oral cavity and pharynx, and of 207 controls [5] found an association with alcohol drinking. Rothman and Keller [6] reanalyzed information on consumption of alcohol and tobacco obtained by Keller and Terris [7]. After stratifying for smoking, the risk for oropharyngeal cancer increased with increasing alcohol consumption at every level of smoking. As found earlier [5], the analysis showed multiplicative interactions between alcohol and tobacco.

Evidence for the role of alcohol and tobacco in cancer of the oral cavity also came from a study in France [8]. The average daily consumption of alcohol was significantly increased in patients with cancer of the tongue, buccal cavity, oropharynx, and hypopharynx. Further case-control studies in Puerto Rico and the United States [9,10] confirmed the role of alcohol in cancer of the oral cavity.

Larynx

Early clinical and occupational studies showed an association between heavy alcohol drinking and laryngeal cancer [11,12]. In most studies of alcoholics, laryngeal cancer is in excess [13,14]. Among male Danish brewery workers, the risk of laryngeal cancer was twice as high as expected [4]. In a number of case-control studies, the role of alcohol and tobacco has been investigated in detail. Wynder et al. [5] found that the risk of laryngeal cancer increased with the amount of whisky taken, even after adjusting for tobacco. In a later study, Wynder et al. [15] confirmed the dose-response relationship, though the increase in risk was less than in the earlier studies.

Studies from the United States, Denmark, and Canada [16-18] confirmed the dual role of alcohol and tobacco in increasing the risk of laryngeal cancer. In nearly all these analyses, the two factors were found to interact in a multiplicative fashion.

Oesophagus

A high prevalence of alcoholism has been generally found among patients with oesophageal cancer [19]. The risk was increased among persons employed in the production or distribution of alcoholic beverages [4,20].
Wynder and Bross [21] found a dose-response relationship between oesophageal cancer and consumption of whisky and beer by smokers of 16-34 cigarettes per day. The risk was approximately 25 times higher among drinkers of 7 or more units of whisky per day, compared to light whisky consumers. A dose-response relationship also emerged among beer consumers.
In a similar study in Paris, Schwartz et al. [8] found average alcohol consumption was significantly higher among patients with oesophageal cancer than among traffic accident victims used as controls. Martinez [10] found a dose-response relationship in a study in Puerto Rico for the risk of oesophageal cancer in relation to daily consumption of alcohol. In a series of studies conducted in France, Tuyns et al. [22,23] found dose-response relationships between the consumption of alcohol after adjustment for tobacco and the risk of oesophageal cancer. The joint effect of alcohol and tobacco was multiplicative with a very high risk among persons who both drank and smoked heavily. There was an indication that the risk of oesophageal cancer might be particularly pronounced for consumers of distillates of apple cider. In a further study, Tuyns [24] examined the risk associated with alcohol consumption among a small number of male and female patients with oesophageal cancer who never smoked. In both sexes, the risk was greater with increasing daily alcohol consumption. A similar association was found in a study in Singapore [25]. In a case-control study of black men in Washington, D.C., Pottern et al. [26] found that the risk was more pronounced among consumers of hard liquor than among consumers of beer (relative risks of 7.3 and 2.7, respectively).

Other Cancer Sites

Stomach

Although there is no indication of increased risk of cancer of the stomach among Finnish alcoholics or Danish brewery workers [4,27], Sundby [28] found a mortality ratio of 1.6 for stomach cancer among alcoholics in Norway. Correlation studies in France and in Japan [29,30] were also suggestive that alcohol may be of aetiological importance in gastric cancer. One case-control study has shown an association between stomach cancer and wine-drinking [31], but other studies of individuals have not given support for such an association [8,32-35].

Colon and Rectum

Breslow and Enstrom [36] found an association between beer sales and rectal cancer in 41 states in the U.S. and in 24 countries. When consumption data for fat were taken into account, the correlation with colon cancer disappeared, while the positive correlation between beer consumption and rectal cancer remained [37]. In Denmark, no increased risk of either colon or rectal cancer was found among brewery workers [4], but a similar study among brewery workers in Ireland showed a doubling of the risk of rectal cancer [38]. A non-significant increased risk of rectal cancer was found in one case-control study by Tuyns et al. [35], and in another case-control study an increased risk for beer consumption in females but not males [39]. In a further case-control study conducted in Australia [40], there was little evidence of an association of any alcoholic beverages with colon cancer, but beer was found to be a risk factor for rectal cancer. The effect was more marked in males than in females, but the relative risks for females were consistent with those for males. The relative risk for the highest consumption levels in quartiles compared to the lowest was approximately 2. The risk of rectal cancer appeared to depend on beer drinking patterns in the previous 15-20 years. Nevertheless, in other case-control studies, either no or only a weak association has been found between alcohol and the risk of colorectal cancer, for the two sites considered together [41,42]. By contrast, in cohort studies in Norway [43] and in Hawaii [44], a dose-response relationship was found between risk of rectal cancer and consumption of alcohol, especially with regard to frequency of beer consumption.

Pancreas

Some studies suggested an association between cancer of the pancreas and alcohol consumption [45,46]. However, most studies of alcoholics have not shown an increased risk of cancer of the pancreas [13,27], nor have cohort studies or case-control studies confirmed an increased risk [4,35,47].

Liver (primary)

In North America and Western Europe, cirrhosis of the liver is mainly related to alcohol consumption. There is a firm association between cirrhosis of the liver and primary liver cancer (PLC) [23]. However, not all studies of alcoholics have shown an increased risk of PLC [14,48]. Among male Danish brewery workers, however, there was a clear association between PLC and cirrhosis of the liver [4]. In Finland, a significant excess of PLC was found among alcohol abusers [27]. Some studies have suggested that PLC may be increased in alcoholics, even in the absence of cirrhosis [49].

Evidence on viral hepatitis and PLC in the alcoholic is accumulating. An increased prevalence of serologic markers of viral hepatitis has been reported in alcoholics [50-55]. Whether this increased incidence of positivity merely reflects the socio-economic status of the alcoholic, whether it is a consequence of increased exposure to hepatitis infection from blood transfusions, or whether it results from enhanced susceptibility to infection remains to be determined.

Brechot et al. [50] evaluated 20 subjects with alcoholic cirrhosis and PLC for evidence of HBV infection. Of these, 16 were tested serologically. Nine out of these 16 had serologic markers of HBV infection. In all 20 subjects with cirrhosis and PLC, the presence of HBV DNA integrated into the genome of the neoplastic liver cells was demonstrated. However, Omata et al. [56] found no difference in the frequency of hepatitis infection in alcoholic cirrhotics with or without PLC at autopsy. Goudeau et al. [57] noted the presence of HBV markers in 31% of 125 asymptomatic alcoholics, 54% of the 163 alcoholics with cirrhosis, and 22% of 46 with PLC. Yarrish et al. [58] reported similar rates of HBV infection in both alcoholic and non-alcoholic subjects with PLC. Of their alcoholic subjects with PLC 88% were seropositive for HBV markers, compared to 69% of non-alcoholic subjects with PLC.

Breast

In most studies which have evaluated an association, it has been found that there appears to be an increased risk of breast cancer in relation to alcohol consumption [59]. There was a positive correlation between alcohol consumption and breast cancer in 41 states in the U.S., but not internationally [36]. A two-fold increase of breast cancer mortality was observed among 2,070 persons admitted to mental hospitals with a diagnosis of alcoholism [60]. Data collected as part of the Third National Cancer Survey in the U.S. showed an increased relative risk of 1.5 for breast cancer from consumption of hard liquor and wine. There was also a dose-response relationship with total alcohol consumption [61]. In a further case-control study, Rosenberg et al. [62] found increased risk of breast cancer for drinkers compared with non-drinkers; the association being evident for beer, wine and spirits. In a case-control study conducted in France, Lé et al. [63] found an increased risk of breast cancer for consumption of alcoholic beverages with meals. The association was significant for beer (relative risk of 2.2 for consumers as compared to non-consumers), and wine (relative risk 1.5). In a cohort study of over 88,000 women from a multiphasic health examination programme, a significant positive trend in the incidence of breast cancer was associated with reported alcohol consumption, though the association was not entirely regular at the highest consumption levels [64]. Similarly, in a 4-year follow-up study of nearly 90,000 U.S. nurses aged 34 to 59, a significant dose-response relationship was found between consumption of alcohol and risk of breast cancer [65]. Among women consuming 5-14 g of alcohol daily (about 3-9 drinks per week), the age-adjusted relative risk of breast cancer was 1.3 (95% CI, 1.0-1.7). For those consuming 15 g of alcohol or more per day, the relative risk was 1.6 (1.3-2.0). Adjustment for known breast cancer risk factors and a variety of nutritional variables did not materially alter this association.

Nevertheless, at least three studies have shown no evidence of an association between alcohol and breast cancer [66,67] or only provided very limited support [68]. Furthermore, in many of the positive studies, nutritional variables could not be fully evaluated. It is therefore possible that increased alcohol consumption may be a marker of other factors which increase the risk of breast cancer.

Summary and Conclusions

Of all the dietary factors shown to increase the risk of cancer, the evidence is strongest for alcohol. Recently, following a thorough evaluation of the available evidence, the International Agency for Research on Cancer [69] found that there is sufficient evidence for the carcinogenicity of alcoholic beverages in humans, and that the occurrence of malignant tumours of the oral cavity, pharynx, larynx, oesophagus and liver is causally related to the consumption of alcohol. There is no indication that the association with drinking is dependent on type of alcoholic beverage.

For cancers of other sites which have been associated with alcohol, the evidence is insufficient to regard these associations as causal, as confounding with other factors has not been fully evaluated.

Cancers of the oral cavity, pharynx, larynx and oesophagus are also causally related to tobacco smoking [70]. The association with alcoholic beverages is independent of tobacco smoking for cancers of these sites, since the risk increases with the amount drunk, irrespective of the level of smoking. An association with drinking has also been observed in lifetime non-smokers in most of the studies where this aspect has been investigated.

REFERENCES

1 De Lint J, Levison T: Mortality among patients treated for alcoholism: a 5-year follow-up. Canad Med Assoc J 1975 (113):385-387

2 Lyon JL, Klauber MR, Gardner JW, Smart CR: Cancer incidence in Mormons and non-Mormons in Utah, 1966-1970. N Eng J Med 1976 (294):129-133

3 Registrar General. Decennial Supplement for England and Wales, 1951. Occupational Mortality, Vol II, Tables. London: HMSO, 1958

4 Jensen OM: Cancer morbidity and causes of death among Danish brewery workers. Int J Cancer 1979 (23):454-463

5 Wynder EL, Bross IJ, Feldmann RM: A study of etiological factors in cancer of the mouth. Cancer 1957 (10):1300-1323

6 Rothman KJ, Keller AZ: The effect of joint exposure to alcohol and tobacco on risk of cancer of the mouth and pharynx. J Chron Dis 1972 (25):711-716

7 Keller AZ, Terris M: The association of alcohol and tobacco with cancer of the mouth and pharynx. Am J Pub Hlth 1965 (55):1578-1585

8 Schwartz D, Lellouch J, Flamant R, Denoix PF: Alcool et cancer. Resultats d'une enquète rétrospective. Rev Fr Etudes Clin Biol 1962 (7):590-604

9 Graham S, Dayal H, Rohrer T et al: Dentition, diet, tobacco and alcohol in the epidemiology of oral cancer. JNCI 1977 (59):1611-1618

10 Martinez I: Factors associated with cancer of the oesophagus, mouth and pharynx in Puerto-Rico. JNCI 1969 (42):1069-1094

11 Kennaway EL, Kennaway NM: A further study of the incidence of cancer of the lung and larynx. Br J Cancer 1947 (1):260-298

12 Kirchner JA, Malkin JS: Cancer of the larynx. AMA Arch Otolaryngol 1953 (5):19-30

13 Monson RR, Lyon JL: Proportional mortality among alcoholics. Cancer 1975 (36):1077-1079

14 Schmidt W, De Lint J: Causes of death of alcoholics. Quart J Stud Alcohol 1972 (33):171-185

15 Wynder EL, Covey LS, Mabuchi K et al: Environmental factors in cancer of the larynx: a second look. Cancer 1976 (38):1591-1601

16 Burch JD, Howe GR, Miller AB, Semincew R: Tobacco, alcohol, asbestos and nickel in the etiology of cancer of the larynx. A case-control study. JNCI 1981 (67):1219-1224

17 Graham S, Mettlin C, Marshall J et al: Dietary factors in the epidemiology of cancer of the larynx. Am J Epidemiol 1981 (113): 675-680

18 Olsen J, Sabroe S, Fasting U: Interaction of alcohol and tobacco as risk factors in cancer of the laryngeal region. J Epid Comm Hlth 1985 (39): 165-168
19 Piquet J,Tison: Alcool et cancer de l'oesophage. Bull Acad Med 1937 (117):236-239
20 Versluys JJ: Cancer and occupation in the Netherlands. Br J Cancer 1949 (3):161-185
21 Wynder EL, Bross IJ: A study of etiological factors in cancer of the esophagus. Cancer 1961 (14):389-413
22 Tuyns AJ, Pequignot G, Jensen OM: Le cancer de l'oesophage en Ille-et-Vilaine en fonction des niveaux de consommation d'alcool et de tabac. Des risques qui se multiplient. Bull Cancer 1977 (64):45-60
23 Tuyns AJ: Alcohol. In: Schottenfeld D, Fraumeni JF (eds) Cancer, Epidemiology and Prevention. Philadelphia: Saunders 1982 pp 293-303
24 Tuyns AJ: Oesophageal cancer in non-smoking drinkers and in non-drinking smokers. Int J Cancer 1983 (32):443-444
25 De Jong JUW, Breslow N, Goh JEH et al: Aetiological factors in oesophageal cancer in Singapore Chinese. Int J Cancer 1974 (13):291-303
26 Pottern LM, Morris LE, Blot WJ et al: Esophageal cancer among black men in Washington DC. I. Alcohol, tobacco and other risk factors. JNCI 1981 (67):777-783
27 Hakulinen T, Lehtimaki L, Lehtonen M, Teppo L: Cancer morbidity among two male cohorts with increased alcohol consumption in Finland. JNCI 1974 (52):1711-1714
28 Sundby P: Alcoholism and Mortality. Oslo: Universitetsforlaget, 1967
29 Audigier JC, Lambert R: Epidemiologie des cancers du tube digestif. Arch Franc Mal Appar Dig 1974 (63):413-432
30 Hirayama T: Epidemiology of stomach cancer. Gann Monogr 1971 (11):3
31 Hoey J, Montvernay C, Lambert R: Wine and tobacco: risk factors for gastric cancer in France. Am J Epidemiol 1981 (113):668-674
32 Acheson ED, Doll R: Dietary factors in carcinoma of the stomach: a study of 100 cases and 200 controls. Gut 1964 (5):126-131
33 Graham S, Scholtz W, Martino P: Alimentary factors in the epidemiology of gastric cancer. Cancer 1972 (30):927-928
34 Haenszel W, Kurihara M, Segi M, Lee RKC: Stomach cancer among Japanese in Hawaii. JNCI 1972 (49): 969-988
35 Tuyns AJ, Pequignot G, Gignoux M et al: Cancers of the digestive tract, alcohol and tobacco. Int J Cancer 1982 (30):9-11
36 Breslow NE, Enstrom JE: Geographic correlations between cancer mortality rates and alcohol-tobacco consumption in the United States. JNCI 1974 (53):631-639
37 Schrauzer GN: Cancer mortality correlation studies. II. Regional associations of mortalities with the consumption of foods and other conditions. Med Hyp 1976 (2):39-49
38 Dean G, MacLennan R, McLoughlin H, Shelly E: The causes of death of blue-collar workers at a Dublin brewery, 1954-1973. Br J Cancer 1979 (40):581-589
39 Miller AB, Howe GR, Jain M et al: Food items and food groups as risk factors in a case-control study of diet and colo-rectal cancer. Int J Cancer 1983 (32):155-161
40 Kune S, Kune GA, Watson LF: 1987. Case-control study of alcoholic beverages as etiological factors: the Melbourne colorectal cancer study. Nutrition and Cancer 1987 (9):43-56
41 Graham S, Dayal H, Swanson M et al: Diet in the epidemiology of cancer of the colon and rectum. JNCI 1978 (61):709-714
42 Dales LG, Friedman GD, Ury HK et al: A case-control study of relationships of diet and other traits to colorectal cancer in American blacks. Am J Epidemiol 1979 (109):132-144
43 Bjelke E: Dietary factors and the epidemiology of cancer of the stomach and large bowel. In: Kasper H (ed) Aktuelle Probleme der klinischen Diatetik. Erkrankungen des Verdauungstraktes. Supplement zu Aktuelle Ernahrungsmedizin. Stuttgart: Georg Thieme Verlag, 1978 pp 10-17
44 Pollack ES, Nomura MY, Heilbrun LK et al: Prospective study of alcohol consumption and cancer. N Eng J Med 1985 (310):617-621
45 Burch CE, Ansari A: Chronic alcoholism and carcinoma of the pancreas; a correlative hypothesis. Arch Intern Med 1968 (122):273-275
46 Cubilla AL, Fitzgerald PJ: Pancreas cancer (non-endocrine): a review. Part II. Clin Bull 1978 (8):143-155
47 MacMahon B, Yen S, Trichopoulos D et al: Coffee and cancer of the pancreas. N Eng J Med 1981 (304):630-633
48 Nicholls P, Edwards G, Kyle E: Alcoholics admitted to four hospitals in England. II General and cause-specific mortality. Quart J Stud Alcohol 1974 (35):841-855
49 Lieber CS, Seitz HK, Garro AJ et al: Alcohol related diseases and carcinogenesis. Cancer Res (39):2863-2886

50 Brechot C, Nalpas B, Courouce A et al: Evidence that hepatitis B virus has a role in liver cell carcinoma in alcoholic liver disease. N Eng J Med 1982 (306): 1384-1387

51 Chevilotte, Durbec G, Gerolami A et al: Interaction between hapatitis B virus and alcohol consumption in liver cirrhosis. Gastroenterology 1983 (85):141-145

52 Gluud C, Gluud B, Aldershville J et al: Prevalence of hepatitis B virus infection in out-patient alcoholics. Infection l984 (l2):72-74

53 Hislop WS, Follet EAC, Bouchier IAD et al: Serological markers of hepatitis B in patients with alcoholic liver disease: a multi-centre survey. J Clin Pathol 1981 (34):1017-1019

54 Mills PR, Rennington TH, Kay P et al: Hepatitis B antibody in alcoholic cirrhosis. J Clin Pathol 1979 (32):778-782

55 Orholm M, Aldershvile J, Tagt-Jensen U et al: Prevalence of hepatitis B virus infection among alcoholic patients with liver disease. J Clin Pathol 1981 (34):1378-1380

56 Omata M, Ashcavai M, Liew C et al: Hepatocellular carcinoma in the USA, etiologic considerations. Gastroenterol 1979 (76):280-287

57 Goudeau A, Maupas P, Dubois F et al: Hepatitis B infection in alcoholic liver disease and primary hepatocellular carcinoma in France. Prog Med Virol 1981 (27):26-34

58 Yarrish RL, Weiner BG, Blumberg BS: Association of hepatitis B virus infection with hepatocellular carcinoma in American patients. Int J Cancer 1980 (26):711-715

59 Graham S: Alcohol and breast cancer. N Eng J Med 1987 (316):1211-1213

60 Adelstein A,White G: Alcoholism and mortality. Population trends. HMSO 1976 (6):7-13

61 Williams RR, Horm JW: Association of cancer sites with tobacco and alcohol consumption and socioeconomic status of patients: interview study from the Third National Cancer Survey. JNCI 1977 (58):525-547

62 Rosenberg L, Slone D, Shapiro S et al: Breast cancer and alcoholic beverage consumption. Lancet 1982 (1):267-271

63 Lé MG, Hill C, Kramar A, Flamant R: Alcoholic beverage consumption and breast cancer in a French case-control study. Am J Epidemiol 1984 (120):350-357

64 Hiatt RA, Bawol RD: Alcoholic beverage consumption and breast cancer incidence. Am J Epidemiol 1984 (120):676-683

65 Willett WC, Stampfer MJ, Colditz GA et al: Moderate alcohol consumption and the risk of breast cancer. N Eng J Med 1987 (316):1174-1180

66 Byers T, Funch DP: Alcohol and breast cancer. Lancet 1982 (1):799-800

67 Webster LA, Layde P, Wingo PA et al: Alcohol consumption and risk of breast cancer. Lancet 1983 (2):724-726

68 Begg CB, Walker AM, Wessen B, Zelen M: Alcohol consumption and breast cancer. Lancet 1983 (1):293-294

69 IARC Monographs on the evaluation of the carcinogenic risk of chemicals to humans. Alcohol Drinking. International Agency for Research on Cancer, Lyon 1988 (in press)

70 IARC Monographs on the evaluation of carcinogenic risk of chemicals to humans. Tobacco Smoking. International Agency for Research on Cancer, Lyon 1986 (38)

Summary: Synthesis and Future Directions

A. B. Miller, F. Berrino, M. Hill, O. M. Jensen, E. Riboli, J. Wahrendorf

Introduction

Of the known causes of cancer, dietary factors collectively contribute to a very large proportion of all potentially preventable cancers. This is probably as true in developing countries as it increasingly appears to be true for the technically advanced countries, though most, but not all, of the data have been derived from the latter. The challenge for those interested in cancer aetiology and prevention is to refine our present knowledge to the stage where appropriate and acceptable recommendations can be made on optimal dietary patterns. Such recommendations must be designed not only to reduce the incidence of cancer of most or several sites, but to prevent adverse changes in the rates of all cancers. At the same time such recommendations must be compatible with those made for the prevention of other dietary associated diseases, especially cardiovascular disease.

Dietary Factors and Cancer Risk

Dietary Fat and Obesity

Of all dietary factors believed to affect cancer incidence, dietary fat has perhaps attracted most interest. This is in part due to the strong correlations noted in international data between the incidence of or mortality from certain cancer sites and estimated population intake of dietary fat, and in part because of observations from animal experimental models. The international correlation studies (ecologic studies) cannot be used to infer causality, but they are useful in raising hypotheses. They may also provide some indication of the range of an effect, which may be difficult to determine within a country if dietary patterns are relatively homogeneous. On the other hand, perhaps particularly with regard to colorectal cancer, animal models have been developed specifically to explore mechanisms potentially relevant to a hypothesis and therefore cannot be used to confirm the validity of that hypothesis.

Most emphasis must therefore be placed on the results of case-control and cohort studies, which, however, with regard to dietary fat and most cancer sites, display much inconsistency. Unfortunately, many of the reported studies were based on inadequate dietary methodology, often with a very indirect assessment of dietary fat intake. In addition, all the case-control studies provide estimates of fat intake which relate to current or recent diet, and which therefore only imperfectly, if at all, reflect diet at the relevant time period for cancer induction. The fact that fat intake is highly correlated with calories makes the evaluation of the association with cancer of each of the two specific factors uncertain.

Epidemiological studies have provided some evidence that dietary fats are a determinant of breast cancer. The association is probably not a simple linear one, since there may be no exposure-effect relationship at high levels of intake. A number of observations suggest that fatty acid composition may be relevant, and that excess saturated fat intake is important in increasing risk.

There is some evidence that prostate cancer is associated with high intake of foods rich in animal fat.

Obesity has been found to be associated with an increased risk of breast cancer in postmenopausal women, though there has been

some inconsistency between the results of different studies. Obesity has been consistently found to be a determinant of endometrial cancer, probably a causal one.
Epidemiological studies do not provide unequivocal evidence for a causal role of dietary fat intake in the aetiology of colorectal and kidney cancer. However, the evidence does not rule out a role for dietary fat since the risk factors identified in terms of food, nutrients, dietary habits and their consequences are all associated to a considerable extent with high fat intake.

Dietary fibre

Most of the methodological problems discussed above for epidemiological studies of dietary fat apply also to studies of dietary fibre. In addition, the methodology for assessment of dietary fibre has undergone marked changes in the past decade, without any final conclusion as to what constitutes dietary fibre, or in some instances, the components of dietary fibre that are potentially relevant in cancer aetiology. Thus dietary data bases, especially in the past, were often inadequate to provide estimates of dietary fibre intake, studies purporting to support the "dietary fibre hypothesis" being dependent on indexes of "fibre-rich foods".
Most of the studies relate to colo-rectal cancer and, with few exceptions, no association has been found for dietary fibre *per se* in case-control studies. Ecologic studies have given inconsistent results. In view of the methodologic difficulties, it would seem prudent neither to conclude that current results reflect the absence of a true association between dietary fibre intake and colo-rectal cancer, nor that a truly protective effect of dietary fibre has just not been detectable by the studies performed to date. Animal studies have not been helpful in clarifying the possible relationship between fibre ingestion and colo-rectal cancer.
However, evidence is accumulating that the incidence of colo-rectal and other cancers (especially stomach and perhaps oesophageal cancer) is reduced in consumers of vegetables and fresh fruit, whose consumption in the daily diet can therefore be encouraged without risk of undesirable side-effects.

Alcohol

Of all dietary factors shown to increase the risk of cancer, the evidence is strongest for alcohol. Although the largest risks relate to cancers shown to be increased by a joint exposure to cigarette smoking (especially oral cavity, pharyngeal and oesophageal cancer, and the parts of the extrinsic larynx directly exposed to alcohol), the evidence is now conclusive that alcohol alone increases the risk of these cancers. There has to be concern, therefore, over the fact that increases in incidence of cancers of these sites have been documented in many countries.
Alcohol consumption is also causally related to primary liver cancer, while the role of alcohol in increasing the risk of colon, rectal and breast cancer is still uncertain. The associations noted for the latter sites may reflect confounding with other causal factors.

Other dietary factors

A host of studies have evaluated the effect of various vitamins, minerals, beverages and other dietary components on the risk of a number of cancer sites. Although many have concluded that specific dietary factors (for example beta-carotene or vitamin C) may be protective against certain cancers, and have inferred that adding such factors to current diet may provide a more acceptable approach to cancer control than dietary change, the current evidence does not justify such an approach. A major difficulty is that the majority of the studies with significant findings were derived from an incomplete assessment of dietary intake, and therefore the investigators were unable to evaluate the possibility that the dietary factor considered was confounded by another, more relevant, dietary factor. Indeed, those few studies that have included complete dietary assessment have in general failed to show that the specific micronutrient under consideration (for example beta-carotene or vitamin C) made an independent contribution once other factors were taken into account. Thus recommendations can not be made for dietary supplementation with any micronutrient on present evidence. Rather, increase in the intake of fresh fruit and vegetables will have the effect of increasing intake of some of the postulated protective factors. Further, intervention trials currently in progress will eventually provide more precise information as to whether supplementation with some micronutrients will reduce cancer risk.

The studies of coffee, tea and artificial sweetener consumption in relation to a number of cancer sites shows no important nor consistent increase in risk of any site.

Of the other factors considered, only for aflatoxin is there conclusive evidence of increase in cancer risk (though only for liver cancer). There is, however, some epidemiological evidence that excess nitrite and/or salt consumption will increase the risk of stomach cancer, while as yet undefined micronutrient deficiencies probably increase the risk of oesophageal cancer.

Methodological Issues in the Investigation of Diet and Cancer in Humans

Many methodological problems have affected the investigation of dietary associations in human cancer, especially with regard to the early studies of dietary fat and fibre.

The methodological factors that should be taken into consideration when planning new research include using a dietary assessment method able to provide information on total energy intake and on major nutrients, adapting the method to local culture and local eating habits, adapting the method to the educational level of the subjects to be investigated, testing the repeatability and the relative validity of the method under field conditions, and adapting food composition tables to food locally consumed. Biochemical markers of nutrient intake should be used when appropriate and feasible, while markers of individual genetic traits may enable subgroups of subjects more or less susceptible to the health effects of particular dietary habits to be identified. Repeated measurements on the same subjects may be considered if the precision of the dietary assessment method or of a biological marker is not satisfactory.

Implications for Food Policies

Science does not exist in a vacuum, yet often the implications of advance in scientific understanding may be missed by those responsible for taking action. In particular, governmental actions taken on economic grounds may have adverse health effects. The agricultural policies of, for example, the European Economic Community, have for some time encouraged the production of fat and alcohol. An increase in fat intake and particularly in saturated fat may specifically effect areas of Southern Europe where some dietary associated cancers are much lower in incidence than in Northern or Western Europe. On the other hand, the recently observed increase in alcohol consumption in Central and Northern Europe may lead to an increase in the incidence of cancers of the upper digestive tract in these areas. There is, therefore, a risk of a major increase in incidence of dietary associated cancers in Europe, other than the decline in stomach cancer already observed. National government policies should be directed to reducing dietary fat and alcohol consumption, as concluded, for example, in the recently implemented Action Programme Against Cancer of the European Community.